Current Concepts in Flexor Tendon Repair and Rehabilitation

Editors

ROWENA MCBEATH
KEVIN C. CHUNG

HAND CLINICS

www.hand.theclinics.com

Consulting Editor
KEVIN C. CHUNG

May 2023 • Volume 39 • Number 2

ELSEVIER

1600 John F. Kennedy Boulevard • Suite 1800 • Philadelphia, Pennsylvania, 19103-2899

http://www.theclinics.com

HAND CLINICS Volume 39, Number 2
May 2023 ISSN 0749-0712, ISBN-13: 978-0-323-94015-3

Editor: Megan Ashdown
Developmental Editor: Hannah Almira Lopez

Hand Clinics (ISSN 0749-0712) is published quarterly by Elsevier Inc., 360 Park Avenue South, New York, NY 10010-1710. Months of publication are February, May, August, and November. Business and Editorial Offices: 1600 John F. Kennedy Blvd., Ste. 1800, Philadelphia, PA 19103-2899. Customer Service Office: 3251 Riverport Lane, Maryland Heights, MO 63043. Periodicals postage paid at New York, NY and at additional mailing offices. Subscription price is $444.00 per year (domestic individuals), $878.00 per year (domestic institutions), $100.00 per year (domestic students/residents), $506.00 per year (Canadian individuals), $1023.00 per year (Canadian institutions), $568.00 per year (international individuals), $1023.00 per year (international institutions), $256.00 (international students/residents), and $100.00 (Canadian students/residents). Foreign air speed delivery is included in all *Clinics* subscription prices. All prices are subject to change without notice. **POSTMASTER:** Send address changes to *Hand Clinics*, Elsevier Health Sciences Division, Subscription Customer Service, 3251 Riverport Lane, Maryland Heights, MO 63043. Customer Service (orders, claims, online, change of address): Elsevier Health Sciences Division, Subscription **Customer Service, 3251 Riverport Lane, Maryland Heights, MO 63043. Tel: 1-800-654-2452 (U.S. and Canada); 314-447-8871 (outside U.S. and Canada). Fax: 314-447-8029. E-mail: journalscustomerservice-usa@elsevier.com (for print support); journalsonlinesupport-usa@elsevier.com (for online support).**

Reprints. For copies of 100 or more of articles in this publication, please contact the Commercial Reprints Department, Elsevier Inc., 360 Park Avenue South, New York, New York 10010-1710. Tel.: 212-633-3874; Fax: 212-633-3820; E-mail: reprints@elsevier.com.

Hand Clinics is covered in *MEDLINE/PubMed (Index Medicus)*, *Current Contents/Clinical Medicine*, *EMBASE/Excerpta Medica*, and *ISI/BIOMED*.

Contributors

CONSULTING EDITOR

KEVIN C. CHUNG, MD, MS
Charles B.G. de Nancrede Professor of Surgery, Professor of Plastic Surgery and Orthopaedic Surgery, Chief of Hand Surgery, Department of Surgery, Section of Plastic Surgery, Michigan Medicine, Assistant Dean for Faculty Affairs, Associate Director of Global REACH, University of Michigan Medical School, Comprehensive Hand Center, University of Michigan, The University of Michigan Health System, Ann Arbor, Michigan, USA

EDITORS

ROWENA MCBEATH, MD, PhD
Attending Hand Surgeon, Philadelphia Hand to Shoulder Center, Assistant Professor, Department of Orthopaedic Surgery, Thomas Jefferson University, Philadelphia, Pennsylvania, USA

KEVIN C. CHUNG, MD, MS
Charles B.G. de Nancrede Professor of Surgery, Professor of Plastic Surgery and Orthopaedic Surgery, Chief of Hand Surgery, Department of Surgery, Section of Plastic Surgery, Michigan Medicine, Assistant Dean for Faculty Affairs, Associate Director of Global REACH, University of Michigan Medical School, Comprehensive Hand Center, University of Michigan, The University of Michigan Health System, Ann Arbor, Michigan, USA

AUTHORS

ROCCO AICALE, MD
Department of Musculoskeletal Disorders, Faculty of Medicine and Surgery, University of Salerno, Baronissi, Italy; Clinica Ortopedica, Ospedale San Giovanni di Dio e Ruggi D'Aragona, Salerno, Italy

CRISTIAN ALETTO, MD
Department of Musculoskeletal Disorders, Faculty of Medicine and Surgery, University of Salerno, Baronissi, Italy; Clinica Ortopedica, Ospedale San Giovanni di Dio e Ruggi D'Aragona, Salerno, Italy

PETER C. AMADIO, MD
Department of Orthopedic Surgery, Mayo Clinic, Rochester, Minnesota, USA

INGA S. BESMENS, MD
Consultant, Department of Plastic Surgery and Hand Surgery, University Hospital Zurich, Zurich, Switzerland

JORDAN BURGESS, BA
Division of Plastic and Reconstructive Surgery, Stanford University Medical Center, Palo Alto, California, USA

RYAN P. CALFEE, MD, MSC
Professor, Department of Orthopedic Surgery, Washington University School of Medicine, St Louis, Missouri, USA

JAMES CHANG, MD
Chair, Division of Plastic and Reconstructive Surgery, Stanford University Medical Center, Chase Hand and Upper Limb Center, Palo Alto, California, USA

DAVID CHOLOK, MD
Division of Plastic and Reconstructive Surgery,
Stanford University Medical Center, Palo Alto,
California, USA

KEVIN C. CHUNG, MD, MS
Charles B.G. de Nancrede Professor of
Surgery, Professor of Plastic Surgery and
Orthopaedic Surgery, Chief of Hand Surgery,
Department of Surgery, Section of Plastic
Surgery, Michigan Medicine, Assistant Dean
for Faculty Affairs, Associate Director of Global
REACH, University of Michigan Medical
School, Comprehensive Hand Center,
University of Michigan, The University of
Michigan Health System, Ann Arbor, Michigan,
USA

ROGER CORNWALL, MD
Clinical Director, Division of Pediatric
Orthopaedics, Department of Orthopedic
Surgery, Director, Hand and Upper Extremity
Surgery Fellowship, Cincinnati Children's
Hospital Medical Center, Cincinnati, Ohio,
USA

LAUREN M. DETULLIO, MOT, OTR/L, CHT
Director, Hand Therapy, Philadelphia Hand to
Shoulder Center, Director, Hand Rehabilitation
Foundation, Philadelphia, USA

PAIGE M. FOX, MD, PhD
Division of Plastic and Reconstructive Surgery,
Stanford University Medical Center, Chase
Hand and Upper Limb Center, Palo Alto,
California, USA

BENJAMIN K. GUNDLACH, MD
Hand Fellow, Philadelphia Hand to Shoulder
Center, Thomas Jefferson University Hospital,
Philadelphia, Pennsylvania, USA

LEILA HARHAUS, MD
Professor and Chair, Department of Hand,
Plastic and Reconstructive Surgery, Burn
Center, BG Trauma Center Ludwigshafen,
Department of Hand and Plastic Surgery,
University of Heidelberg, Heidelberg,
Germany

SALLY JO, MD
Department of Orthopedic Surgery,
Washington University School of Medicine, St
Louis, Missouri, USA

DONALD H. LALONDE, FRCSC
Professor of Surgery, Dalhousie University,
Saint John, New Brunswick, Canada

TOMOYUKI KUROIWA, MD, PHD
Department of Orthopedic Surgery, Mayo
Clinic, Rochester, Minnesota, USA

**NICOLA MAFFULLI, MD, MS, PhD, FRCS
(Orth)**
Department of Musculoskeletal Disorders,
Faculty of Medicine and Surgery, University of
Salerno, Baronissi, Italy; Clinica Ortopedica,
Ospedale San Giovanni di Dio e Ruggi
D'Aragona, Salerno, Italy; Queen Mary
University of London, Barts and the London
School of Medicine and Dentistry, Centre for
Sports and Exercise Medicine, Mile End
Hospital, London, England; Keele University,
Faculty of Medicine, School of Pharmacy and
Bioengineering, Guy Hilton Research Centre,
Stoke-on-Trent, England

ROWENA MCBEATH, MD, PhD
Attending Hand Surgeon, Philadelphia
Hand to Shoulder Center, Assistant Professor,
Department of Orthopaedic Surgery, Thomas
Jefferson University, Philadelphia,
Pennsylvania, USA

ANDREW J. MILLER, MD
Philadelphia Hand to Shoulder Center,
Assistant Professor, Department of
Orthopaedic Surgery, Thomas Jefferson
University, Philadelphia, Pennsylvania, USA

GIOVANNI MUNZ, MD
Consultant, Azienda Ospedaliera Careggi:
Azienda Ospedaliero Universitaria Careggi,
Surgery and Microsurgery of the Hand, Firenze,
Italy; Unit of Hand Surgery, Santo Stefano
Hospital, Prato, Italy

FRANCESCO OLIVA, MD
Department of Musculoskeletal Disorders,
Faculty of Medicine and Surgery, University of
Salerno, Baronissi, Italy; Clinica Ortopedica,
Ospedale San Giovanni di Dio e Ruggi
D'Aragona, Salerno, Italy

A. LEE OSTERMAN, MD
Philadelphia Hand to Shoulder Center,
Professor, Department of Orthopaedic Surgery,
Thomas Jefferson University, Philadelphia,
Pennsylvania, USA

ZHANG JUN PAN, MD
Chief, Hand Surgery, Yixing City Hospital,
Yixing, Jiangsu, China

SARAL J. PATEL, MBBS, MS
Philadelphia Hand to Shoulder Center,
Philadelphia, Pennsylvania,
USA

SARVNAZ SEPEHRIPOUR, MD
Birmingham Women's and Children's National
Health Service Foundation Trust, Steelhouse
Lane, Birmingham, England, United
Kingdom

SARAH E. SASOR, MD
Assistant Professor, Department of Plastic
Surgery, Medical College of Wisconsin,
Milwaukee, Wisconsin, USA

TERRI M. SKIRVEN, BSCOT, OTR/L, CHT
Director Emeritus, Hand Therapy, Philadelphia
Hand to Shoulder Center

BRIAN W. STARR, MD
Section of Plastic Surgery, The University of
Michigan Health System, Ann Arbor, Michigan,
USA

JIN BO TANG, MD
Professor and Chair, Department of Hand
Surgery, The Hand Surgery Research Center,
Affiliated Hospital of Nantong University,
Nantong, Jiangsu, China

DAVID S. ZELOUF, MD
Attending Physician, Philadelphia Hand to
Shoulder Center, Thomas Jefferson University
Hospital, Philadelphia, Pennsylvania, USA

Contributors

ZHANG JUN FAN, MD
Chief Hand Surgery, Wujing, Dr. Shenzhen,
Futian, Fujian, China

SARAL J. PATEL, MBBS, MS
Philadelphia Hand to Shoulder Center,
Philadelphia, Pennsylvania,
USA

SARVNAZ SEPEHRIPOUR, MD
Birmingham Women's and Children's National
Health Service Foundation Trust, Steelhouse
Lane, Birmingham, England, United
Kingdom

EFRAH E. SADOK, MD
Assistant Professor, Department of Plastic
Surgery, University of Wisconsin,
Milwaukee, Wisconsin, USA

TERINA HSIANG, DSOT, OTR/L, CHT
Clinical Therapist, Hand Therapy, Philadelphia
Hand to Shoulder Center

BRIAN W. STARR, MD
Section of Plastic Surgery, The University of
Michigan Health System, Ann Arbor, Michigan
USA

JIN BO TANG, MD
Professor and Chair, Department of Hand
Surgery, The Hand Surgery Research Center,
Affiliated Hospital of Nantong University,
Nantong, Jiangsu, China

DAVID S. ZELOUF, MD
Attending Physician, Philadelphia Hand to
Shoulder Center, Thomas Jefferson University
Hospital, Philadelphia, Pennsylvania, USA

Contents

Principles of Tendon Structure, Healing, and the Microenvironment   119

Rowena McBeath and Kevin C. Chung

> Tendon is a strong viscoelastic tissue, responsible for conducting force from muscle to bone. In the hand, flexor tendons course through fibro-osseous sheaths, composed of an intricate tenosynovium and fibrocartilaginous pulley system. After flexor tendon laceration, changes occur in tendon force transduction as well as vascularity, affecting tendon healing on a tissue and cellular level. Tendon healing occurs through intrinsic and extrinsic mechanisms, which in combination with local anatomy, can predispose to adhesion formation. Understanding the relationship between microenvironmental cues and tendon healing on the cellular and tissue level will improve our knowledge and treatment of flexor tendon injuries.

General Principles of Flexor Tendon Repair   131

Sally Jo and Ryan P. Calfee

> Flexor tendon repair techniques and rehabilitation have advanced tremendously in the past 50 years. However, the attributes of the ideal tendon repair articulated by Dr Strickland in 1995 hold true today. The ideal repair requires sutures easily placed in the tendon, secure suture knots, a smooth juncture of the tendon ends, minimal gapping, least interference with tendon vascularity, and sufficient strength throughout healing. When accomplished, the modern flexor tendon repair is a stout repair, sufficient for early mobilization and intrinsic tendon healing.

Flexor Tendon Repair Techniques: M-Tang Repair   141

Jin Bo Tang, Zhang Jun Pan, Giovanni Munz, Inga S. Besmens, and Leila Harhaus

> The authors present the methods and outcomes from six institutes where M-Tang repairs with early active flexion exercise are used for zone 2 digital flexor tendon repair. The authors had close to zero repair ruptures, and few digits needed tenolysis. The excellent to good results are generally between 80% and 90%. In the pandemic period, less stringent therapy supervision might have allowed some patients to move too aggressively, with repair ruptures not seen before the pandemic in one institute. In Nantong, Yixing, and Saint John, the rupture incidence is zero to 1%. In Florence and Heidelberg, the rupture incidence was 3%.

Surgical Considerations for Flexor Tendon Repair: Timing and Choice of Repair Technique and Rehabilitation   151

Sarah E. Sasor and Kevin C. Chung

> Flexor tendon injuries are common and occur mostly due to penetrating trauma. Surgical repair is required for complete tendon lacerations, and many techniques exist. This article reviews the principles of tendon structure, function, healing, and anatomy. Repair techniques are discussed in detail for each flexor tendon zone. Postoperative rehabilitation greatly influences outcomes, and several protocols are described.

Video content accompanies this article at http://www.hand.theclinics.com.

WALANT has generated many changes that have improved flexor tendon repair and reconstruction in the last 10 years. Seeing awake unsedated educable patients move repaired reconstructed tendons during the surgery has changed how we do surgery and therapy in many ways for the better. This article offers many tips on how to get better results in using these new techniques with the help of WALANT.

Over the years, various physical and chemical/biological methods of inhibiting adhesion formation have been developed, focusing on how to suppress healing around the tendon and not inhibit healing within the tendon. Unfortunately, however, these methods are accompanied by drawbacks, both large and small, and no absolute antiadhesion method capable of maintaining tendon repair strength has yet been developed. Recent innovations in biomaterials science and tissue engineering have produced new antiadhesion technologies, such as barriers combined with cytokines and cells, which have improved outcomes in animal models, and which may find clinical relevance in the future.

Rehabilitation after flexor tendon repairs is a challenging process. The repaired tendon must be simultaneously protected from disruption and moved in a controlled fashion to prevent restrictive adhesion formation. Although measures are necessary to protect the repaired structures, early controlled motion is required to enhance healing and function. Appropriate intervention at the correct phase of healing is based on an understanding of tendon healing and the factors that influence it. Coordination and communication between the surgeon and therapist is essential. Tendon injuries can profoundly affect hand function, and appropriate rehabilitation is essential to preserve function to the fullest extent possible.

Chronic injury to the flexor tendon system of the hand remains a challenging problem for the hand surgeon to treat. Both single- and two-stage techniques remain important in the reconstruction of the flexor tendon deficient digit. Modern advances include the use of allograft composites that aim to reduce the time and donor-site morbidity compared with conventional autograft techniques. Regardless of technique, restoring a gliding tendon-pulley system with a functional arc of motion is the primary goal of flexor tendon reconstruction.

 Video content accompanies this article at http://www.hand.theclinics.com.

Complications in flexor tendon repair are common and include tendon rupture, adhesion formation, and joint contracture. Risk factors include preexisting conditions, gross contamination, concurrent fracture, early unplanned loading of the repaired tendon, premature cessation of splinting, and aggressive early active range of motion protocols with insufficient repair strength. Rupture of a repaired tendon should be followed by early operative exploration, debridement, and revision with a four-core strand suture and nonbraided epitendinous suture. Wide-awake flexor tenolysis should be considered when adhesion formation results in the plateaued range of motion, and passive motion exceeds active motion. Two-staged reconstruction is recommended when injury results in excessive scaring, joint contracture, or an incompetent pulley apparatus.

HAND CLINICS

SERIES OF RELATED INTEREST:

Clinics in Plastic Surgery
www.plasticsurgery.theclinics.com

Orthopedic Clinics of North America
www.orthopedic.theclinics.com

Clinics in Sports Medicine
www.sportsmed.theclinics.com

THE CLINICS ARE AVAILABLE ONLINE!
Access your subscription at:
www.theclinics.com

Preface

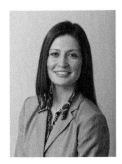 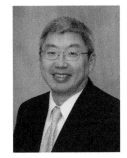

Rowena McBeath, MD, PhD   Kevin C. Chung, MD, MS
Editors

Tension of the musculoskeletal system—force transmission enabling function, creation, and existence—is maintained by tendons. To all of us, tendons are essential to every facet of life, whether it be performing basic needs of living or creating music and art. To us as physicians and surgeons of the hand and upper extremity, tendons allow us to take care of our patients.

Tendon injury is ubiquitous. Yet, despite their familiar hierarchical anatomy and well-studied cellular and molecular architecture, predictable surgical outcomes remain elusive. We are fortunate to have the most prescient and creative minds in our specialty. It was our quest in this issue to define our current understanding of the basic biological mechanisms of tendon structure and function, emphasize those factors essential to tendon repair and healing, present treatment possibilities when repair and healing processes go awry, as well as detail the evolution of the mechanical environment conducive to the best healing outcomes. We feel this special issue has accomplished our task.

Similar to what has existed before us, as well as what will follow us, this issue is a snapshot in time. After Sterling Bunnell presented his fraught results after intrasynovial tendon repair, tendon repair in zone 2 was not attempted for many years. We hope to use the knowledge presented in this issue to inspire questions and techniques that will improve our outcomes after tendon repair, and thus further enhance the care of our patients.

Rowena McBeath, MD, PhD
Philadelphia Hand to Shoulder Center
Department of Orthopaedic Surgery
Thomas Jefferson University
834 Chestnut Street
Philadelphia, PA 19107, USA

Kevin C. Chung, MD, MS
Professor of Surgery
Department of Surgery
Section of Plastic Surgery
University of Michigan
1500 East Medical Center Drive
2130 Taubman Center, SPC 5340
Ann Arbor, MI 48109, USA

E-mail addresses:
rmcbeath@handcenters.com (R. McBeath)
kecchung@med.umich.edu (K.C. Chung)

Hand Clin 39 (2023) xi
https://doi.org/10.1016/j.hcl.2023.02.001
0749-0712/23/© 2023 Published by Elsevier Inc.

Principles of Tendon Structure, Healing, and the Microenvironment

Rowena McBeath, MD, PhD[a,b,*], Kevin C. Chung, MD, MS[c]

KEYWORDS

- Tenocyte • Vinculae • Fibril • Phenotype • Extrinsic • Intrinsic • Tenosynovium

KEY POINTS

- Tendons are composed of cells (tenocytes) in collagen-rich extracellular matrix and are responsible for force transduction from muscle to bone.
- Flexor tendons of the hand pass through fibro-osseous sheaths composed of tenosynovium as well as fibrocartilaginous pulleys.
- This anatomic structure of flexor tendons in the hand predisposes to adhesion formation after repair.
- Healing capacity of tendon depends on cues in the tendon microenvironment including oxygen levels and force transmission.

INTRODUCTION

In the musculoskeletal system, "form follows function." The concept that musculoskeletal tissues develop from the tensile and compressive forces that they conduct was proposed centuries ago by the anatomist and surgeon Julius Wolff with respect to bone remodeling, in that bone will adapt to the loads under which it is placed.[1] Although a soft tissue, tendon is strong in that it is capable of transmitting equal forces as bone, through tensile in principle more so than compressive mechanisms.[2] The ability of tendon to transmit such loads—important to the hand with respect to maximizing heavy grip as well as fine dexterous movement—is due to its gross and cellular anatomic structure.

Flexor Tendon Zones of the Hand

In 1983, the Committee of Tendon injuries cochaired by Kleinert and Verdan agreed on anatomic nomenclature regarding flexor tendon zones as presented by Eaton and Weilby.[3] In this report, flexor tendons of the hand were divided into 5 zones: zone I (distal to proximal interphalangeal joint [PIPJ]), zone II (A1 to PIPJ), zone III (palm), zone IV (carpal tunnel), and zone V (wrist and forearm; **Fig. 1**A). In the thumb, these zones include zone I (distal to interphalangeal joint [IPJ]), zone II (A1), zone III (thenar eminence), and with zones IV and V the same as for fingers.[3] These zones persist today and have undergone further subclassification in zones I,[4] II,[5] and V[6] (**Fig. 1**B, **Table 1**).

Although the zones of flexor tendon injury in the hand have remained relatively unchanged during the last few decades, decision-making has evolved concerning whether to repair or reconstruct zone II injuries, as well as timing, method of repair, sheath preservation or excision, and repair of one or both tendons.[7] Although zone II injuries—of all zones—have the most unpredictable outcomes due to adhesion formation, most surgeons agree that flexor tendon injuries should be repaired by a surgeon familiar with the anatomy of the fibro-osseous sheath.

[a] Philadelphia Hand to Shoulder Center, Philadelphia, PA, USA; [b] Department of Orthopaedic Surgery, Thomas Jefferson University, Philadelphia, PA, USA; [c] Department of Surgery, Section of Plastic Surgery, University of Michigan, 1500 East Medical Center Drive 2130 Taubman Center, SPC 5340, Ann Arbor, MI 48109, USA
* Corresponding author. 834 Chestnut Street, Suite G-114 Philadelphia, PA 19107.
E-mail address: rmcbeath@handcenters.com

Hand Clin 39 (2023) 119–129
https://doi.org/10.1016/j.hcl.2023.01.002
0749-0712/23/© 2023 Published by Elsevier Inc.

A

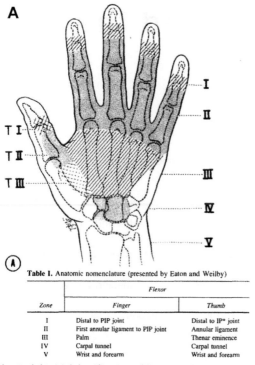

Table I. Anatomic nomenclature (presented by Eaton and Weilby)

	Flexor	
Zone	Finger	Thumb
I	Distal to PIP joint	Distal to IP* joint
II	First annular ligament to PIP joint	Annular ligament
III	Palm	Thenar eminence
IV	Carpal tunnel	Carpal tunnel
V	Wrist and forearm	Wrist and forearm

B

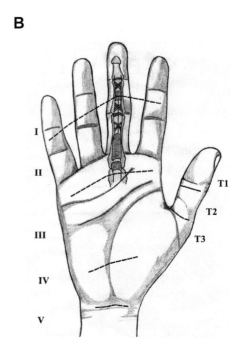

Fig. 1. (*A*) Initial classification of flexor tendon zones in the hand and fingers. (*B*) Further classification of flexor tendon zones in the hand. (*From [A]* Kleinert HE and Verdan C. Report of the Committee on Tendon Injuries. Journal of Hand Surgery 1983. 8 (5 pt 2): 794-798; and [*B*] Venkatramani H, Varadharajan V, Bhardwaj P, Vallurupalli A, Sabapathy SR. Flexor tendon injuries. J Clin Orthop Trauma. 2019;10(5):853-861. https://doi.org/10.1016/j.jcot.2019.08.005.)

Tenosynovium and Pulley System: Fibro-Osseous Sheath

Classic anatomic studies of the hand and fingers revealed what we know today as the structure of

Table 1
Flexor tendon zones of the hand

	Region	Subclassification
Zone 1	Distal to FDS insertion	1a: from bone[4] 2a: from 1a to distal edge A4 pulley[4] 3a: beneath or proximal to A4 pulley[4] 1p: pull-off (avulsion)[4]
Zone II	FDS insertion to A1	2a: proximal A4 to C2[5] 2b: C2 to C1[5] 2c: deep to A2[5] 2d: deep to A1[5]
Zone III	A1 to distal aspect of flexor retinaculum	
Zone IV	Carpal tunnel under flexor retinaculum	
Zone V	Proximal to the flexor retinaculum[6]	

Abbreviation: FDS, flexor digitorum superficialis.

the finger flexor sheath and pulley system.[8–15] In a series of cadaveric studies, Doyle injected the synovial sheaths of 61 cadaveric fingers with methylene blue. Using a microscope, they documented the structure of 5 annular pulleys and 3 cruciform pulleys and a tenosynovial sheath, which we identify today as the fibro-osseous sheath (**Fig. 2**A and B).[16] The synovial sheath ("membranous" portion) was described as a tube sealed at both ends, with the pulleys ("retinacular" portion) overlaying the synovium at discrete intervals, with the floor of the pulleys being the volar plates and volar surfaces of the phalanges. Finger flexion was achieved without bowstringing owing to the broader pulleys (A2 and A4) localized between joints, whereas narrow (A1, A3, A5, and cruciform) were over the joints, with segmental pulley arrangement with synovial windows in between.[16] One unique finding in the flexor tendons of the digits is that the fibro-osseous sheath provides function through form—increased gliding provided by the tenosynovium, coupled with mechanically optimized range of motion through pulley composition and position.

More than mechanical function, the role of the tenosynovium in maintaining tendon homeostasis through diffusion from the synovial fluid was first

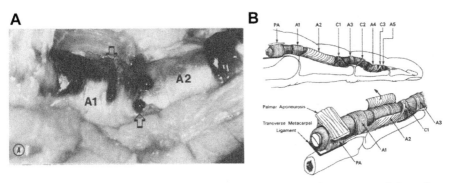

Fig. 2. (*A*) Cadaveric finger injection with methylene blue, demonstrating the anatomy of the pulleys and teno-synovial sheath. (*B*) The fibro-osseous sheath. (*From* Doyle JR, Blythe W. Macroscopic and functional anatomy of the flexor tendon sheath. J Bone Joint Surg 1974: 56A: 1094; with permission.)

proposed in 1907 and has been demonstrated by multiple investigators.[17,18] Most definitively, Manske and colleagues[19] used a hydrogen washout technique in a chicken flexor tendon model to examine the ability of the tenosynovium to provide tendon nutrition. A oxygen–hydrogen gaseous mixture was administered to the chickens and measured using platinum electrodes on the intact tendon. Two treatment groups were then created; in one case, the tendon was isolated from its synovium but the vasculature remained intact. In the other group, the vinculae were divided but the synovium left intact. The gaseous mixture was administered to each group and then measured; surprisingly, none of those tendons isolated from the synovium demonstrated hydrogen uptake, whereas all of those tendons with synovium intact but vinculae divided demonstrated near-normal hydrogen uptake (**Fig. 3**).[19] These results emphasized the importance of the synovium to maintaining tendon homeostasis. Other investigators also demonstrated the ability of tendons to survive in the absence of discrete vasculature by implanting transected tendons into the synovial pouch of the rabbit knee,[20–23] as well as demonstrating tendon survival and healing in in vitro explant culture.[24] These studies delineated the ability of tendon to survive in the absence of discrete vasculature in a synovial or other fluid environment.

It is seen from the complex yet elegant structure of the fibro-osseous sheath that in the setting of flexor tendon injury, mechanical friction between suture of the lacerated tendon and the sheath, increased by swelling and vascular ingrowth after repair, will contribute to decreased tendon excursion, subsequent adhesion formation, and onset of stiffness. It is this conundrum—of balancing the strength of the tendon repair with ease of passage through the sheath despite the propensity for adhesion formation—that led Dr J Phillip Matthews to conclude that "Of all the problems which

face the surgeon dealing with hand injuries, few have proved as difficult to solve as that of the flexor tendon which has been severed within the digital sheath."[25] In his studies of the effect of simple tenotomy versus tenotomy coupled with surgical repair in a rabbit model, Matthews found the presence of adhesion formation in both cases, irrespective of injury level along the sheath (**Fig. 4**).[25] Furthermore, examination of tendon specimens via silver iodine perfusion revealed adhesion formation within the first 3 weeks in both conditions, with cut-out of the suture from the tendon in the repair group, leading to the conclusion that the circulation through the tendon may be adversely affected by the initial injury itself as well as the repair technique.[25] Similarly, Matthews and Richards also noted excision of the synovial sheath (as well as suture of partially lacerated tendon and immobilization) as a factor contributing to adhesion formation in rabbits.[26] These studies emphasized the importance of damage to the synovial sheath to adhesion formation.

With respect to the pulley component of the fibro-osseous sheath, it was demonstrated by Peterson and colleagues[27] in a human cadaver model that retaining both A2 and A4 pulleys was necessary for near-normal digital flexion. More recently, multiple studies have demonstrated good outcomes after zone II flexor tendon repair with pulley venting, coupled with a strong repair and early postoperative mobilization.[5]

Vascular System: Vinculae

Tendons were originally regarded as avascular structures[28,29]; however, classic cadaveric injection studies led anatomists such as Berkenbusch to observe that (1) the tendon is vascularized from palmar vessels derived from vinculae within the digital sheath, and at the osseous insertion,

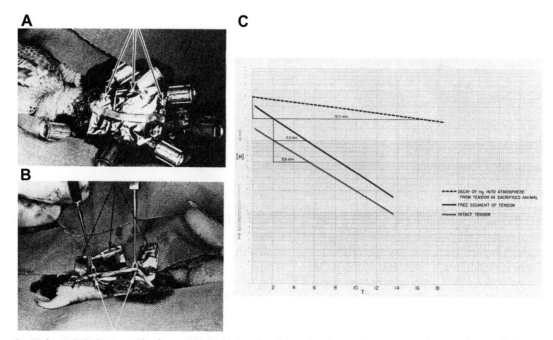

Fig. 3. (*A* and *B*) Photograph of experimental setup for determination of hydrogen washout technique in chicken flexor tendons, with (*A*) the vinculae divided yet the synovium left intact, or (*B*) with the vinculae intact (see *arrows*) but the synovium stripped. (*C*) Graphical representation of hydrogen measurements from tendon with vinculae divided "free tendon" compared with normal "intact tendon." (*From* Manske PR, Whiteside LA and Lesker PA. Nutrient pathways to flexor tendons using hydrogen washout technique. J Hand Surg Am 1978 3(1): 32-36; with permission.)

(2) both the profundus and the superficialis tendons have consistent areas of avascularity more commonly in adults than in children, and (3) most vessels remain on the tendon surface; those entering the substance ended in loops rather than form a network of capillaries.[30,31]

Similarly, classic anatomic studies of the hand and fingers identified tendon vasculature.[32–43] Using India-ink injection of fresh cadaveric human hands, Ochiai and colleagues[42] identified 4 transverse communicating braches of the digital arteries that entered the fibro osseous canal

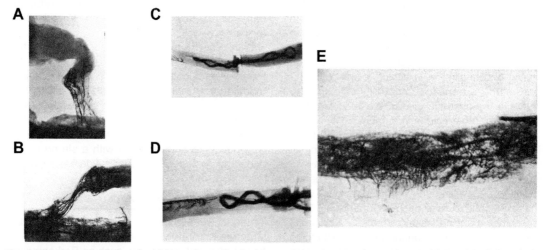

Fig. 4. Photomicrographs of rabbit tendon adhesion formation, after simple tenotomy: (*A*) 3 weeks (*B*) 8 weeks, and (*C–E*) after tenotomy and tendon repair: (*C*) 2 days, (*D*) 4 days, and (*E*) 3 weeks. (*From* Matthews JP. Vascular changes in flexor tendons after injury and repair: an experimental study. Injury. 1977;8(3):227-233; with permission.)

through openings in the pulleys: the distal transverse, interphalangeal transverse, proximal transverse, and branch to vinculum longus superficialis (VLS; **Fig. 5**). All these branches contributed to the vinculae, which were short and long folds of the mesotenon (see **Fig. 5**). Short vinculae, vinculum breve superficialis originated from the membranous volar plate of the PIPJ, whereas the vinculum breve profundus originated from the distal two-thirds of the middle phalanx; the short vinculae were consistent in all fingers (see **Fig. 5**). The long vinculae varied among fingers, and included VLS (3 types: radial, ulnar, absent), which originated from the base of the proximal phalanx, and vinculum longus profundus (5 types: distal, middle, mixed, proximal, absent), which originated from the FDS (see **Fig. 5**).

Although multiple studies delineated the vascular supply to the flexor tendon system, the importance of vinculae to tendon homeostasis and nutrition was debated for many years. Tendon vascularity is necessary because experiments wrapping tendons resulted in avascularity and subsequent tendon necrosis.[43–45] From these anatomic studies and others, it is seen that the vascular supply to tendon is delicate yet deliberate, with vessel pattern influenced by the presence or absence of pulleys. Poor vascularity was demonstrated in the A2 and A4 pulley areas, and good vascularity was demonstrated in the areas of the cruciform pulleys and membranous sheath.[32] Although vascular input to the tendon seems necessary for tendon health, the role of the vasculature to tendon homeostasis is still unclear.

Many investigators proposed the role of tendon vasculature to adhesion formation. Indeed, another predisposing factor for adhesion formation results from rapid vessel ingrowth and increased inflammatory growth factors including transforming growth factor beta 2 (TGFb2) and fibroblast growth factor (FGF). Restoring vascularity after tendon repair remains a delicate balance. Understanding the behavior of tendon tissue and cells to vascular ingrowth and subsequent oxygen levels represents the next frontier of understanding tendon healing.

Tendon Structure and Stages of Tendon Healing

Tendon is a hierarchical structure composed of cells (tenocytes) embedded in a dense extracellular matrix. Tendon extracellular matrix is composed mostly of collagen type Ia1, with small amounts of noncollagenous proteins including proteoglycans.[46] The visible unit structure of tendon is a fascicle, which often contributes to its gross striated appearance, covered by a thin filmy connective tissue known as endotenon. Tendon is composed of groups of collagen fascicles, separated by endotenon, and covered with a similar loose connective tissue known as the epitenon. Vascular supply to the tendon occurs via vessels in the endotenon and epitenon (**Fig. 6**).[46]

The anatomic and microscopic structure of tendon dictates its behavior under stress. Tendon fascicles are composed first of 3 polypeptide chains in a helical pattern, forming tropocollagen. Five tropocollagen molecules cross-linked together form microfibrils, which together form fibrils, then fascicles. This fiber-based structure has tendon viscoelastic properties that influences strain, rate of strain, loading direction, and location.[46] Under slow initial loading, tendon stiffens with increasing strain, resulting from collagen fibrils.[46] Linear stress–strain is then reached, with failure occurring at strain of 10%[46] (see **Fig. 6**).[47,48] Tendon stiffness is also sensitive to location and loading direction, with the greatest stiffness in the direction of the fibers.

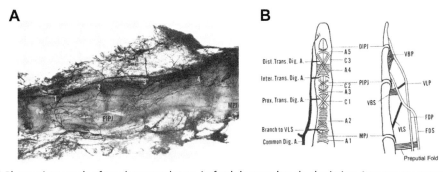

Fig. 5. (A) Photomicrograph of tendon vasculature in fresh human hands, depicting 4 transverse communicating branches from the common digital arteries: (1) distal transverse artery, (2) interphalangeal transverse digital artery, (3) proximal transverse digital artery, and (4) branch to the VLS. (B) A graphical representation of vinculae in the human finger. (*From* Ochiai N, Matsui T, Miyaji N, Merklin RJ, Hunter JM. Vascular anatomy of flexor tendons. I. Vincular system and blood supply of the profundus tendon in the digital sheath. J Hand Surg Am. 1979;4(4):321-330; with permission.)

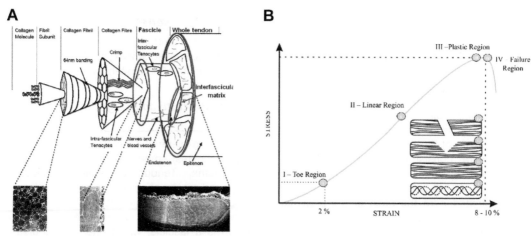

Fig. 6. (*A*) The hierarchical microorganization and macroorganization of tendon. (*B*) The mechanism by which tendon accommodates force. I, intact tendon withstands force in the toe region; II, stretched tendon accommodates force in the linear region; III, partially damaged tendon accommodates force in the plastic region; and IV, failure to accommodate force occurs in the failure region. (*From* [*A*] Thorpe CT, Clegg PD, Birch HL. A review of tendon injury: Why is the equine superficial digital flexor tendon most at risk? Equine Veterinary Journal 2010;42:174-180. https://doi.org/10.2746/042516409X480395; and [*B*] de Cassia Marqueti R, Vieira de Sousa Neto I, Reichert Barin F, et al. (2019) Exercise and Tendon Remodeling Mechanism. Tendons. IntechOpen. DOI: 10.5772/intechopen.79729. © 2019 The Author(s). Licensee IntechOpen. This chapter is distributed under the terms of the Creative Commons Attribution 3.0 License, which permits unrestricted use, distribution, and reproduction in any medium, provided the original work is properly cited.)

Early investigators noted poor healing capacity of tendons,[49] which was thought to be due to decreased cellularity of the tendon.[50] In observations of tendon healing, Bunnell[51] and Garlock[52] noticed the development of adhesions at tendon laceration sites, which were assumed to come from the periphery. Further investigations by Peacock[53] delineated 3 phases to tendon repair: (1) Immediate migration of peripheral cells into the wound site to provide increased vascularity and fibroblasts ("Inflammatory" phase, 24 hours to 7 days),[54] (2) Protein and collagen aggregate formation ("proliferation" phase, 3 days to 4 weeks),[55] (3) Remodelling because of biophysical forces: controlled tension and enzymatic biochemical activity ("remodelling" phase, 4 weeks to months) (**Fig. 7**).[56] These phases have been observed in animal models of intrasynovial and extrasynovial tendon healing.[56]

Initial studies noted that flexor tendon healing occurred through intrinsic and extrinsic mechanisms,[55] with contributions from each depending on the phase of healing. Initially, the inflammatory phase occurs from predominantly extrinsic mechanisms, with influx of inflammatory cells (predominantly neutrophils) resulting in increases of interleukin (IL)-1b, IL-6, and IL-8 (**Fig. 7**).[56,57] Cells at the injury site also release growth factors including: basic fibroblast growth factor (bFGF) (found in fibroblasts and inflammatory cells surrounding the healing site in the tendon sheath),[58]

bone morphogenic protein (elevated early in tendon healing),[59] connective tissue growth factor (elevated during the first 21 days),[60] insulin growth factor-1 (found after 4 to 8 weeks, during formation and remodeling),[61] platelet-derived growth factor (found in healing tendons and persisting more than 6 months postinjury),[62] transforming growth factor b (found throughout the course of tendon healing),[63,64] and vascular endothelial growth factor (with increased activity during the proliferative and remodeling phases)[65] (see **Fig. 7**).[56] Interestingly, these same factors involved in tendon healing also contribute to adhesion formation.[66] Multiple studies have investigating blocking growth factors via antibody-targeted or gene-targeted means; however, the ability to improve intrinsic tendon healing without extrinsic adhesion formation remains elusive.

Tendon Healing and Mechanical Force

Bunnell famously identified injury to the intrasynovial flexor tendon as "no man's land" due to the propensity for adhesion formation after repair,[51] and for many years, attempts at tendon repair in this zone were abandoned.[31] Subsequently multiple investigators, in their quest to improve outcomes, studied the effects of tendon repair, the synovium, and the role of immobilization to adhesion formation. Using a rabbit model, Matthews and Richards found 3 factors that affected adhesion formation

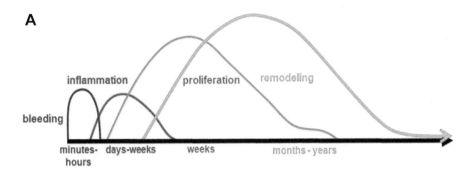

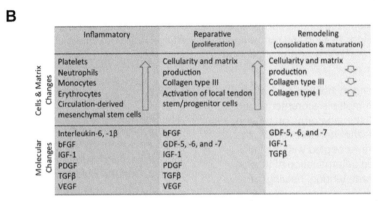

Fig. 7. (*A*) The phases of tendon healing. (*B*) Chart of growth factors present in stages of tendon healing. (*From* [*A*] Schulze-Tanzil GG, Delgado-Calcares M, Stange R, Wildemann B, Docheva D. Tendon healing: a concise review on cellular and molecular mechanisms with a particular focus on the Achilles tendon. Bone Joint Res. 2022;11(8):561-574; and [*B*] Docheva D, Müller SA, Majewski M, Evans CH. Biologics for tendon repair. Adv Drug Deliv Rev. 2015;84:222-239; with permission.)

after tendon repair: (1) suture of a lacerated tendon, (2) excision of the tendon sheath, and (3) immobilization after tendon repair.[26] In their studies, extrasynovial tendon repair followed by immobilization resulted in intrinsic healing, with minimal adhesions. However, when coupled with sheath excision, tendon repair and immobilization resulted in dense adhesions.[26]

Other investigations into the role of the synovial environment on tendon healing examined the effects of mechanical force through altered postoperative motion protocols. In their investigations of flexor tendon healing in a canine model, Gelberman and colleagues[67–69] discovered passive motion after tendon repair resulted in a smooth gliding surface, decreased adhesion formation, and enhanced tensile strength (**Fig. 8**). This finding suggested that motion in and of itself decreases adhesion formation and increases repair quality, although applied force greater than that supported by the repair can lead to tendon rupture.[70] Subsequently, multiple postoperative motion protocols after human flexor tendon repair using passive[71] and active[72,73] motion demonstrated improved clinical outcomes. Currently, most

tendon repairs applied that active postoperative motion protocols.[5]

Given that tendon is a mechanoactive tissue, multiple basic biochemical studies have studied the role of mechanical force and tendon viability, function and gene expression. Maeda and colleagues,[74] in their examination of cyclic loads on tenocytes, found increased expression of collagen type III mRNA in rat tenocytes and increased growth factor concentration in response to mechanical loading. Recently, more attention has been devoted to characterizing the mechanical environment of tenocytes, their cytoskeleton[75] and their relationship with surrounding cells via cell-cell contacts and gap junctions.[76] These results support the evolving concept that mechanical force, aside from maintaining tendon tissue health, affects regulation of differential gene expression.

Tendon Healing and the Oxygen Microenvironment

There has been much interest in the tendon oxygen microenvironment and the effect of this

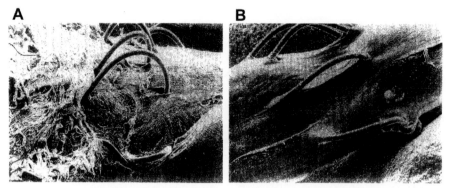

Fig. 8. Scanning electron micrographs of lacerated and sutured canine flexor tendons. (*A*) Immobilized tendon postrepair at 10 days. (*B*) Mobilized tendon postrepair at 42 days. (*From* Gelberman RH, Vande Berg JS, Lundborg GN, Akeson WH. Flexor tendon healing and restoration of the gliding surface. An ultrastructural study in dogs. J Bone Joint Surg Am. 1983;65(1):70-80; with permission.)

microenvironment on tendon healing and adhesion formation. Although multiple aforementioned studies[26,68] determined the anatomy of tendon vasculature before and after tendon repair, the role of tendon vasculature—coupled with the intrasynovial environment—on determination of tendon oxygen concentration and tendon healing continues to be investigated.

Recently, further characterization of the intrasynovial and extrasynovial tendon and its microenvironment has been performed in animal models. Although the intrasynovial tendon has been shown to be relatively avascular,[67] Shen and colleagues[77] recently demonstrated altered extracellular matrix and inflammatory markers in intrasynovial versus extrasynovial tendon, suggesting that the decreased vascularity in the avascular zone in canines affects the tendon phenotype. In this study, there were increased proteoglycans and decreased inflammatory and metabolic responses in the intrasynovial tendon after repair, again supporting improved healing in extrasynovial versus intrasynovial tendons.[77]

Although the exact oxygen concentration in tendon tissue is unknown, it is estimated to be between 1% and 5%, much lower than that in the atmosphere (21% O_2).[78] Hypoxic culture of multiple cell types has been shown to decrease senescence and increase proliferation capacity.[79–81] In our studies of human tenocytes in hypoxia (1% O_2), we discovered increased fibrochondrocyte and mineralized fibrochondrocyte characteristics, suggesting that the oxygen microenvironment affects tenocyte phenotype.[75] This effect depends on intracellular signals responsible for force transmission, suggesting that the tenocyte phenotype and tendon homeostasis depend on both oxygen tension as well as mechanotransduction to maintain cell and tissue health.

SUMMARY

Investigations into the macroscopic, microscopic, and molecular anatomy of flexor tendons and their tenosynovium have resulted in a thorough understanding of the flexor tendon macroenvironment in the hand. Despite these advances, difficulties persist: consistent successful outcomes after intrasynovial flexor tendon repair are difficult to obtain due to adhesion formation. Causes of adhesion formation include mechanical barriers to gliding, as well as an uncontrolled and unbalanced extrinsic and intrinsic healing responses. Although the healing response has been characterized as consisting of a cascade of cells and growth factors, difficulty persists in controlling the tendon healing response for effective intrinsic healing with minimal extrinsic adhesion formation. This imbalance may be due to the effects of the local oxygen and tension microenvironment on the tenocyte phenotype.

DECLARATION OF INTERESTS

National Institutes of Health (R. McBeath, K.C. Chung), book royalties from Wolters Kluwer and Elsevier (K.C. Chung), and a research grant from Sonex to study carpal tunnel outcomes (K.C. Chung).

REFERENCES

1. Wolff J 'Zur Lehre von der Fracturenheilung' (On the Theory of Fracture Healing), 1873, translated by Heller MO, Taylor WR, Aslanidis N, et al., (2010) Clin Orthop Relat Res 468: 1052–5.
2. Maganaris CN, Narici MV. Mechanical properties of tendons. In: Maffulli N, Renström P, Leadbetter WB, editors. Tendon injuries. London: Springer; 2005. https://doi.org/10.1007/1-84628-050-8_2.

3. Kleinert HE, Verdan C. Report of the Committee on Tendon Injuries. J Hand Surg 1983;8(5 pt 2):794–8.

4. Moiemen NS, Elliot D. Primary flexor tendon repair in zone 1. J Hand Surg 2000;25B(1):78–84.

5. Tang JB. Indications, methods, postoperative motion and outcome evaluation of primary flexor tendon repairs in Zone 2. J Hand Surg 2007; 32E:118–29.

6. Sabapathy SR, Elliot D. Complex injuries to the flexors in the hand and forearm. In: Cheema TA, editor. Complex injuries of the hand. London: JP Medical Publishers; 2014.

7. Venkatramani H, Varadharajan V, Bhardwaj P, et al. Flexor tendon injuries. Journal of Clinical Orthopaedics and Trauma 2019;10:853–61.

8. Doyle JR, Blythe W. Macroscopic and functional anatomy of the flexor tendon sheath. J Bone Joint Surg 1974;56A:1094.

9. Verdan CE. Half a century of flexor-tendon surgery, current status and changing philosophies. J Bone Joint Surg 1972;54A:472–91.

10. Barton NJ. Experimental Study of optimal location of flexor tendon pulleys. Plast Reconstr Surg 1969;43: 125–9.

11. de la Caffiniere JY. Anatomie fon ctionnelle de la poulie proximal des doigts. Arch Anat Pathol 1971; 19:357–66.

12. Schneider LH, Hunter JM. Flexor tendons – late reconstruction. In: Green DP, editor. Operative hand surgery. New York: Churchill Livingstone; 1982. p. 1423.

13. Lundborg G, Myrhage R. The vascularization and structure of the human digital tendon sheath as related to flexor tendon function. Scand J Plast Reconstr Surg 1977;11:195–203.

14. Manske PR, Lesker PA. Palmar aponeurosis pulley. J Hand Surg 1983;8:259–63.

15. Strauch B, de Moura W. Digital flexor tendon sheath: an anatomic study. J Hand Surg 1985;10A:785–9.

16. Kleinert HE, Lubahn JD. Current state of flexor tendon surgery. Ann Chir Main 1984;3:7–17.

17. Arai H. Die blutgefasse der Sehnen, 434. Wiesbaden: Anatomische Hefte; 1907. p. 363–82.

18. Potenza AD. Critical evaluation of flexor tendon healing and adhesion formation within artificial digital shealths. J Bone Joint Surg 1963;45A:1217–33.

19. Manske PR, Whiteside LA, Lesker PA. Nutrient pathways to flexor tendons using hydrogen washout technique. J Hand Surg Am 1978;3(1):32–6.

20. Lundborg G. Experimental flexor tendon healing without adhesion formation – A new concept of tendon nutrition and intrinsic healing mechanisms. A preliminary report. J Hand Surg Br Vol 1976;8(3): 235–8.

21. Lundborg G, Rank F. Experimental intrinsic healing of flexor tendons based upon synovial fluid nutrition. J Hand Surg 1978;3(1):21–31.

22. Lundborg G, Holm S, Myrhage R. The role of the synovial fluid and tendon sheath for flexor tendon nutrition. An experimental tracer study on diffusional pathways in dogs. Scand J Plast Reconstr Surg 1980;14:99–107.

23. Lundborg G, Hansson H-A, Rank F, et al. Superficial repair of severed flexor tendons in synovial environment – An experimental study on cellular mechanisms. J Hand Surg 1980;5(5):451–61.

24. Gelberman RH, Manske PR, Vandeberg JS, et al. Flexor tendon repair in vitro: a comparative histologic study of the rabbit, chicken, dog and monkey. J Orthop Res 1984;2:39–48.

25. Matthews JP. Vascular changes in flexor tendons after injury and repair: an experimental study. Injury 1977;8:227–33.

26. Matthews P, Richards H. Factors in the adherence of flexor tendon after repair: an experimental study in the rabbit. J Bone Joint Surg Br 1976;58:230–6.

27. Peterson WW, Manske PR, Bollinger BA, et al. Effect of pulley excision on flexor tendon biomechanics. J Orthop Res 1986;4(1):96–101.

28. Kolliker A, Busk G, Huxley T, editors. Manual of human histology. London: Printed for the Syndenham Society; 1853.

29. Sappey MPC. Recherches sur les vaisseaux et les nerfs des parties fibreuses et fibro-cartilagineuses. Comptes Rendus Hebdomadaires des Sbeances de L'Acadbemie des Sciences 1866;62:1116–8.

30. Berkenbusch H. Die Blutversorgung der Beugeschen der Finger. Nachrichten der Koniglichen Gesellschaft der Wissenschaften 1887;14:403–6.

31. Manske PR. Flexor tendon healing. J Hand Surg 1988;13B(3):237–45.

32. Doyle JR. Anatomy of the finger flexor tendon sheath and pulley system. J Hand Surg 1988;13A(4): 473–84.

33. Mayer L. The physiological method of tendon transplantation. Surg Gynecol Obstet 1916;22:183.

34. Edwards DAW. The blood supply and lymphatic drainage of tendons. J Anat 1946;80:147.

35. Brockis JG. The blood supply of the flexor and extensor tendons of the fingers in man. J Bone Joint Surg 1946;35:131.

36. Peacock EE Jr. A study of the circulation in normal tendons and healing graft. Ann Surg 1959;149:415.

37. Smith JW. Blood supply of tendons. Am J Surg 1965; 109:272.

38. Chaplin DM. The vascular anatomy within normal tendons, divided tendons, free tendon grafts and pedicle tendon grafts in rabbits. A microradioangiographic study. J Bone Joint Surg 1973;55:1191.

39. Leffert RD, Weiss C, Athanasoulis CA, et al. The vincula. J Bone Joint Surg 1974;56:1191.

40. Caplan HS, Hunter JM, Merklin RJ, et al. Intrinsic vascularization of flexor tendons. AAOS symposium

on tendon surgery in the hand. St Louis (MO): The CV Mosby Co; 1975. p. 48.

41. Lundborg G, Myrhage R, Rydevik B, et al. The vascularization of human flexor tendons within the digital synovial sheath region – structural and functional aspects. J Hand Surg 1977;2:417.

42. Ochiai N, Matsui T, Miyaji N, et al. Vascular anatomy of flexor tendons. I. Vincular system and blood supply of the profundus tendon in the digital sheath. J Hand Surg 1979;4(4):321–30.

43. Weckesser EC, Shaw BW. A comparative study of various substances for the prevention of adhesions about tendons. Surgery 1949;25:361–9.

44. Chaplin DM. The vascular anatomy within normal tendons, divided tendons, free tendon grafts and pedicle tendon grafts in rabbits. A microradioangiographic study. J Bone Joint Surg Br 1973;55:369–89.

45. Tempfer H, Traweger A. Tendon vasculature in health and disease. Front Physiol 2015;6(330):1–7.

46. Voleti PB, Buckley MR, Soslowsky LJ. Tendon healing: Repair and regeneration. Annu Rev Biomed Eng 2012;14:47–71.

47. Marqueti RD, Neto IV, Barin FR, et al. Exercise and Tendon remodeling mechanism. From Tendons, Edited by Hasan Sozen, published by IntechOpen, pp1-20.

48. Thorpe CT, Udeze CP, Birch HL, et al. Capacity for sliding between tendon fascicles decreases with ageing in injury prone equine tendons: a possible mechanism for age-related tendinopathy? Eur Cell Mater 2013;25:48–60.

49. Bier A. Beobachtungen uber regeneration beim Menschen. Deutsche med. Wohnschr. 1917. 43: 705, 833, 864, 897, 925, 1025, 1057, 1121, 1249.

50. Salomon A. Keinische und experimentello Untersuchungen veber Heilung Ven Sehnenverlctzungen Insbesondere Innerhalb der fibreuses Sehnenscheiden. Archiv Fuer Klinische Chirurgie 1924; 129:397–430.

51. Bunnell S. Repair of tendons in the fingers. Surg Gynecol Obstet 1922;35:88–97.

52. Garlock JH. Repair of wounds of the flexor tendons of the hand. Ann Surg 1926;83:111–2.

53. Peacock EE. Biological principles in the healing of long tendons. Surg Clin North Am 1965;45:461–76.

54. Potenza AD. Mechanisms of healing of digital flexor tendons. J Hand Surg Br Vol 1969;1(1):40–1.

55. Lindsay WK, Thomson HG. Digital flexor tendons: an Experimental study, Part I. The significance of each component of the flexor mechanism in tendon healing. Br J Plastic Surg 1960;12:289–319.

56. Docheva D, Muller SA, Majewski M, et al. Biologics for tendon repair. Adv Drug Deliv Rev 2015;84:222–39.

57. Manning CN, Havlioglu N, Knutsen E, et al. The early inflammatory response after flexor tendon healing: a gene expression and histological analysis. J Orthop Res 2014;32(5):645–52.

58. Chang J, Most D, Thunder R, et al. Molecular studies in flexor tendon wound healing: the role of basic fibroblast growth factor gene expression. J Hand Surg Am 1998;23:1052–8.

59. Heisterbach PE, Todorov A, Fluckiger R, et al. Effect of BMP-12, TGFb1 and autologous conditioned serum on growth factor expression in Achilles tendon healing. Knee Surg Sports Traumatol Arthrosc 2012;20:1907–14.

60. Chen CH, Cao Y, Wu YF, et al. Tendon healing in vivo: gene expression and production of multiple growth factors in early tendon healing period. J Hand Surg Am 2008;33:1834–42.

61. Dahlgren LA, Mohammed HO, Nixon AJ. Temporal expression of growth factors and matrix molecules in healing tendon lesions. J Orthop Res 2005;23:84–92.

62. Chan BP, Fu SC, Qin L, et al. Supplementation-time dependence of growth factors in promoting tendon healing. Clin Orthop Relat Res 2006;448:240–7.

63. Chang J, Thunder R, Most D, et al. Studies in flexor tendon wound healing: neutralizing antibody to TGF-beta1 increases postoperative range of motion. Plast Reconstr Surg 2000;105:148–55.

64. Natsu-ume T, Nakamura N, Shino K, et al. Temporal and spatial expression of transforming growth factor-beta in the healing patellar ligament of the rat. J Orthop Res 1997;15:837–43.

65. Petersen W, Unterhauser F, Pufe T, et al. The angiogenic peptide vascular endothelial growth factor (VEGF) is expressed during the remodeling of free tendon grafts in sheep. Arch Orthop Trauma Surg 2003;123:168–74.

66. Juneja SC, Schwarz EM, O'Keefe RJ, et al. Cellular and molecular factors in flexor tendon repair and adhesions: a histological and gene expression analysis. Connect Tissue Res 2013;54:218–26.

67. Gelberman RH, Amiel D, Gonsalves M, et al. The influence of protected passive mobilization on the healing of flexor tendons: A biochemical and micrangiographic study. J Hand Surg Br Vol 1981;13(2):120–8.

68. Gelberman RH, Woo SL, Lothringer K, et al. Effects of early intermittent passive mobilization on healing canine flexor tendons. J Hand Surg 1982;7(2):170–5.

69. Gelberman RH, Vandeberg JS, Lundborg GN, et al. Flexor tendon healing and restoration of the gliding surface. An ultrastructural study in dogs. J Bone Joint Surg 1983;65S:70–80.

70. Titan AL, Foster DS, Chang J, et al. Flexor tendon: development, healing, adhesion formation, and contributing growth factors. Plast Reconstr Surg 2019;144(4):639e–47e.

71. Duran RJ, Houser RG, Coleman CR, et al. A preliminary report in the use of controlled passive

motion following flexor tendon repair in zone II and III. J Hand Surg 1976;1:79.

72. Becker H. Primary repair of flexor tendons in the hand without immobilization – preliminary report. J Hand Surg Br Vol 1978;10(1):37–47.

73. Brunelli G, Vigasio A, Brunelli F. Slip-knot flexor tendon suture in zone II alloweing immediate mobilization. J Hand Surg Br Vol 1983;15(3):352–8.

74. Maeda E, Shelton JC, Bader DL, et al. Differential regulation of gene expression in isolated tendon fascicles exposed to cyclic tensile strain in vitro. J Appl Physiol (1985) 2009;106:506–12.

75. McBeath R, Edwards RW, O'Hara BJ, et al. Tendinosis develops from age- and oxygen tension- dependent modulation of Rac1 activity. Aging Cell 2019; 18(3):e12934.

76. Theodossiou SK, Murray JB, Schiele NR. Cell-cell junctions in developing and adult tendons. Tissue Barriers 2020;8(1):e1695491.

77. Shen H, Yoneda S, Sakiyama-Elbert SE, et al. Flexor tendon injury and repair: the influence of synovial environment on the early healing response in a canine model. J Bone Joint Surg Am 2021;103(9): e36.

78. Fehrer C, Brunauer R, Laschober G, et al. Reduced oxygen tension attenuates differentiation capacity of human mesenchymal stem cells and prolongs their lifespan. Aging Cell 2007;6(6):745–57.

79. Ejtehadifar M, Shamsasenjan K, Movassaghpour A, et al. The effect of hypoxia on mesenchymal stem cell biology. Adv Pharm Bull 2015;5(2):141–9.

80. Zhang J, Wang JHC. Human tendon stem cells better maintain their stemness in hypoxic culture condition. PLoS One 2013;8(4):e61424.

81. Schulze-Tanzil GG, Delgado Caceres M, Stange R, et al. Tendon healing: a concise review on cellular and molecular mechanisms with a particular focus on the Achilles tendon. Bone Joint Res 2022;11(8): 561–74.

General Principles of Flexor Tendon Repair

Sally Jo, MD, Ryan P. Calfee, MD, MSc*

KEYWORDS

• Flexor tendon • Repairs • Zone II • Principles • Laceration • Outcomes

KEY POINTS

• Flexor tendon repairs require both precise repairs and dedication to rehabilitation to achieve optimal results.
• For active motion rehabilitation, flexor tendon repairs require a minimum of four core suture strands.
• Following flexor tendon repair, gapping must remain under 3 mm for the tendon to accrue normal strength.

HISTORY OF FLEXOR TENDON REPAIR

Repair of flexor tendon injuries in the hand is a relatively modern practice.[1] For much of history, these injuries were treated nonoperatively due to the belief that repair consistently led to poor outcomes. Free tendon grafting and primary repair became more common in the 1850s. However, Sterling Bunnell's famous pronouncement of the area between the distal palmar crease and the proximal phalanx as a "no-man's land" recognized the difficulty in restoring a functional digit after surgery.[2,3]

Mason and Allen[4] reported a significant loss of tensile strength at the repair site immediately after repair and immobilization of extra-synovial flexor tendons due to "softening of the tissues and diminution in holding power for the suture." This casted doubt on the durability of flexor tendon repairs. Not until the 1980s was early motion in combination with a stout repair at time zero recognized as key to the early accrual of strength at the repair site. Early motion promotes intrinsic healing by tenocytes rather than by the ingrowth of nearby cells and vessels that create adhesions.[5–7] Today, primary repair followed by early rehabilitation continues to be the treatment of choice for acute flexor tendon injuries, although complications such as stiffness and repair rupture still occur.

PREOPERATIVE EXAMINATION

Like all penetrating trauma, visual assessment first notes the location, size, and contamination of soft-tissue wounds. It is essential to realize that even seemingly small and apparently superficial lacerations over the volar wrist or fingers can lacerate flexor tendons. Radiographs assist in evaluating for any fracture or retained foreign bodies.

During visual inspection, the resting posture of the digits is evaluated. In an uninjured hand, there is a cascade of increasing finger flexion from the index to the small finger. This cascade will be disrupted by a flexor tendon injury (**Fig. 1**). The tenodesis effect of increasing finger flexion with wrist extension should also be assessed. Squeezing the distal forearm can accentuate this effect as it brings the fingers into a more flexed posture. The digit and palm proximal to the injured digit should be palpated for any areas of bulk, which could indicate retracted tendon ends. Typically, the only palpable tendon end is the flexor digitorum profundus (FDP) when caught on the A2 pulley or in the palm proximal to A1.

Next, the neurovascular status of each digit is assessed. Sensation quantified by two-point discrimination on the radial and ulnar borders of the digit is critical to detecting any concomitant nerve injury. Vascular injury is assessed by

Department of Orthopedic Surgery, Washington University School of Medicine, 660 S Euclid Avenue, Campus Box 8233, St. Louis, MO 631, USA
* Corresponding author.
E-mail address: calfeer@wustl.edu

Hand Clin 39 (2023) 131–139
https://doi.org/10.1016/j.hcl.2022.08.014

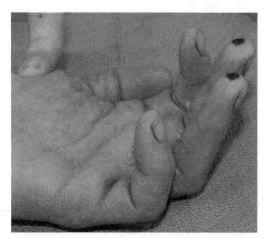

Fig. 1. This left hand shows the loss of normal resting tension in the middle and ring fingers due to FDP lacerations. Note the extended DIP joints that are asymmetric with those of the index and small fingers.

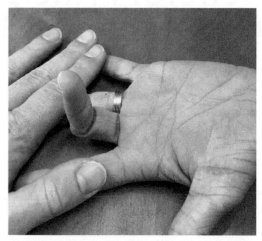

Fig. 3. Active testing for FDS integrity requires blocking other digits in extension to eliminate pull through from the FDP.

checking capillary refill, pulp space turgor, and Allen testing. Doppler ultrasound and fingertip pulse oximeters can supplement evaluations.

Finally, active tendon flexion is evaluated in each digit. The FDP tendon is tested by the examiner holding the middle phalanx in extension and asking the patient to flex the distal interphalangeal (DIP) joint (**Fig. 2**). Active flexion at the DIP signifies an intact FDP tendon. The flexor digitorum superficialis (FDS) tendon is isolated by the examiner holding all other digits in full extension and asking the patient to flex at the PIP joint of interest (**Fig. 3**). Holding the other digits in extension prevents the shared muscle belly of the FDP tendons from firing, and the free digit will flex at the PIP joint only if the FDS tendon is intact. Flexor pollicis longus (FPL) tendon integrity is noted by active interphalangeal (IP) flexion in the thumb. Weakness or

pain with active flexion can signify partial laceration of the tendon.

Flexor tendon injuries are then documented by zones as treatment implications can differ for each zone (**Fig. 4**). Zone I spans from the insertion of the FDP tendon on the distal phalanx to the

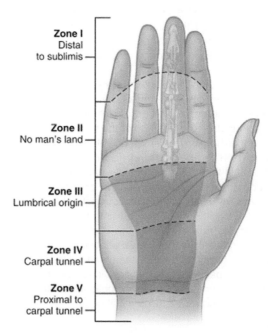

Fig. 4. Flexor zones of hand. Designated zones on flexor surface of hand are helpful because treatment of tendon injuries may vary according to level of severance. (*From Azar FM, Beaty JH, Canon DL. Flexor and Extensor Tendon Injuries. In: Campbell's Operative Orthopaedics. Philadelphia: Elsevier; 2021:3454–3455; with permission.*)

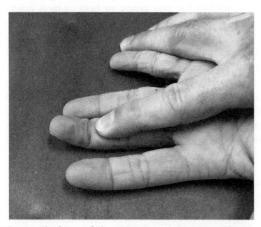

Fig. 2. Blocking of the PIP joint while asking the patient to flex the DIP joint to test integrity of the FDP tendon.

insertion of the FDS tendon on the middle phalanx. Zone II includes the A1 pulley at the distal palmar crease to the insertion of the FDS tendon at the end of the A4 pulley. Zone II is unique in that there are two tendons filling the synovial sheath in this area. There is both the FDS tendon, which divides into radial and ulnar slips in the middle of the A2 pulley, and the FDP tendon, which emerges superficially past the Camper Chiasm. These tendons must glide adhesion-free in a tight pulley system to produce the best outcomes. Zone III is defined from the distal aspect of the transverse carpal ligament to the insertion of the FDS tendon. Zone IV is the zone of the carpal tunnel, and zone V is the area of the forearm proximal to the carpal tunnel. Skin lacerations are only a rough guide to the level of tendon injury. When fingers are lacerated while gripping, the tendon laceration is located substantially more distal than the skin injury.

REPAIRS IN ZONE I

Injuries in zone I are sustained either through direct tendon laceration or the more common avulsion secondary to forced extension of a flexed distal phalanx. Leddy and Packer categorized these avulsion injuries based on the presence of associated fracture and the degree of tendon retraction. Generally, injuries with more FDP retraction should be repaired with more urgency as these tend to be associated with significant retraction of the tendon and disruption of the vincula containing the extrinsic blood supply.[8,9]

Repair of zone I injuries requires securing the tendon end to the distal phalanx. A mid-lateral or zig-zag (Bruner) incision can be made with each finishing obliquely over the pulp space distally. Suture techniques vary from classically described two-strand suture pullout technique to multistrand grasping or locking sutures being used (**Fig. 5**). The sutures are frequently passed with a Keith

straight needle either along the volar periosteum of the distal phalanx to the fingertip or through the distal phalanx exiting the nail plate distal to the germinal matrix. The suture is then tied over a button (**Fig. 6**). Buttons are removed in the office 6 weeks postoperatively. With increasing core strands the sutures are typically then cut flush with the nail at the time of button removal as opposed to being pulled out. Alternatively, suture anchors can provide direct fixation into the distal phalanx. Clinical results remain comparable between the two groups of fixation methods.[10]

Significant retraction of the proximal tendon stump can complicate repair. A proximal counter-incision in the palm may prove necessary to retrieve the tendon. Once identified, the tendon end can be held with a provisional suture and passed using a tendon passer, looped malleable wire, or pediatric feeding tube to deliver the suture through the intended path. Combined swelling of the injured tendon end and shrinking of the A4 pulley create substantial difficulty in passing the tendon back to its insertion.

Injuries in zone I tend to have superior clinical outcomes compared with zone II injuries, as avulsion injuries primarily require stability, and good outcomes are not as reliant on smooth gliding of tendon over the adjacent FDS tendon. Recently though, a retrospective cohort study of 26 patients highlighted the unlikelihood of restoring a normal DIP joint and concluded that those patients treated with surgery were not substantially improved over those that did not undergo tendon repair.[11]

A particular complication associated with FDP repair is the quadrigia effect, which describes the inability to flex fully at the unaffected digits when the injured FDP tendon is shortened or over-advanced. The excursion of the uninjured digits will be limited by the amount of excursion of the

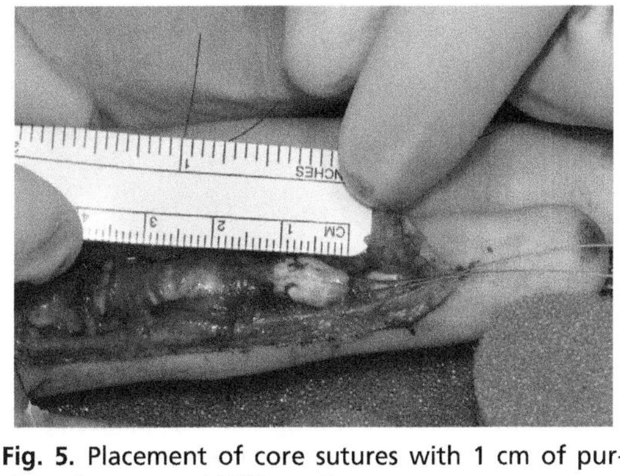

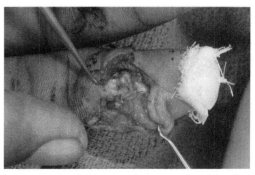

Fig. 5. Placement of core sutures with 1 cm of purchase for a zone I FDP repair.

Fig. 6. Repair of a zone I FDP laceration using a button at the fingertip that allows approximation of tendon ends when the distal FDP stump is too short for primary repair.

shortest tendon that pulls the shared FDP muscle belly of the middle, ring, and small fingers.

The authors do not pursue reconstruction of isolated FDP injuries that present in a delayed fashion. In these situations, any painful mass of FDP tendon in the distal palm may be excised, which routinely improves comfort. If the lack of tension in the DIP joint results in hyperextension impairing function, then we would offer DIP arthrodesis or FDP tenodesis to the DIP volar plate.

REPAIRS IN ZONE II

Flexor tendon injuries are most common in zone II,[12] and post-surgical outcomes in this area are the most variable. The ultimate goal of zone II repair is to optimize repair strength sufficiently for early postoperative rehabilitation. Early motion while maintaining a gap of less than 3 mm[13] at the repair site is necessary for the accrual of tensile strength via intrinsic tendon healing. Early motion also counters the increasing resistance to tendon motion associated with longer periods of immobilization.[14–16] Given the approximate 34 N of force imparted when actively flexing digits, the ideal repair will withstand 50 N of force and heal with gapping of less than 3 mm.[13]

Variations in surgical technique and their influence on the mechanical properties at the repair site are well studied. Key variables include core suture strand number,[17,18] caliber,[19] and purchase, suture technique (eg, modified Kessler technique),[20] epitendinous suture purchase,[21] and locking versus grasping loop configurations. A minimum of 4 core suture strands is necessary for early active rehabilitation and increases loads to failure and decreases risks of adhesion formation and reoperation.[18,20,22] Core suture placement of 7 to 10 mm from the cut edge ensures sufficient tendon purchase.[23] Immaculate tissue handling is critical to preventing adhesion formation, as emphasized by Bunnell.[24]

Repair of zone II injuries is performed through a mid-lateral or Bruner incision. The traumatic wound can be incorporated into the incision. The senior author (RPC) prefers mid-lateral incisions which provide a robust soft-tissue coverage over the flexor tendons (**Fig. 7**). In a mid-lateral approach, the ipsilateral neurovascular bundle is carefully dissected away from the flap being raised allowing it to be retracted dorsally. Next, a window in the fibro-osseous sheath is made and the tendon stumps are identified. Although traditional teaching recommends a routine opening of the sheath from the distal A2 pulley to the proximal A4 pulley, we do not recommend that. We would

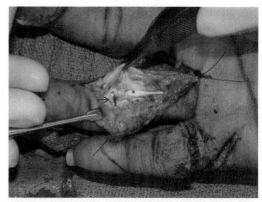

Fig. 7. Mid-lateral approach to zone II flexor tendon laceration showing robust soft-tissue flaps and broad exposure afforded by this approach. Distal FDP stump marked with arrow and FDS slips partially lacerated (stars).

examine the tendon sheath while flexing the IP joints to see where the distal FDP reaches. If the distal FDP cannot reach at least 1 cm proximal to A4, we would release A4 to perform the repair. Related to this, Tang discusses releasing parts of the A2 and A4 pulleys in order to prevent the repair site from catching.[25] Biomechanical studies have shown that partial release of A2 and A4 pulleys does not result in any significant mechanical disadvantage.[25–27] However, when releasing the whole A4, it is critical that A3 and likely the cruciate pulleys are left intact to prevent bowstringing. Retracted stumps can be milked distally. An additional incision may need to be made proximally to retrieve the proximal tendon stump. At our institution, a 3-0 or 4-0 looped nonabsorbable braided suture is used to complete a 4- to 8 strand core suture repair. Then a running epitendinous suture is applied circumferentially to smooth out the edges of the repaired tendon stumps and to increase the tensile strength of the construct (**Fig. 8**).

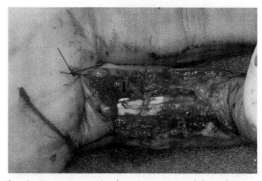

Fig. 8. Zone II repair showing minimal bunching at repair site (*thin arrow*) and at core suture purchase area (*wide arrow*).

Generally, zone II repairs are recommended within a week of injury, and sooner if there is neurovascular compromise. Delay risks greater retraction of the tendon ends and collapse of the pulley system making the repair more difficult. Basic science evidence also supports repair within days of injury.[28] Reconstruction is considered if the patient presents in a delayed fashion such that direct repair is not possible due to irreversible scarring of the pulley sheath or excessive repair tension anticipated to produce either a digit flexion contracture or quadrigia.

REPAIRS IN ZONES III–V

In zones III through V, the flexor tendons are no longer encased in a fibro-osseous sheath. Therefore, the concern for adhesion formation is less with repairs in these zones and early rehabilitation is not as important as in zone II. Another important anatomic consideration in these zones is the proximity of nerves and vessels to the flexor tendons making concomitant neurovascular injury common (**Fig. 9**).

Concomitant injury to neurovascular structures, such as the deep and superficial palmar arches, common digital nerves, deep motor branch of the ulnar nerve, and the motor branch of the median nerve are frequent in zone III. In zone III, Bruner incisions extend traumatic lacerations and injured structures are addressed from deep to superficial. For flexor tendon injuries in the distal portion of zone III, the A1 pulley may be released to prevent the repair site from catching on the pulley. For flexor tendon injuries in the proximal part of zone III, the carpal tunnel can be released to retrieve the injured tendon ends and visualize

injured structures. The results of flexor tendon repair in zone III are generally considered to be better than those of zone II repair due to the decreased risk of scarring that limits tendon gliding.[29]

Zone IV is the zone of the carpal tunnel. An injury to the median nerve and flexor tendons in this zone is colloquially termed "spaghetti wrist." The FDS and FDP tendons lie deep to the median nerve in this zone. A careful assessment of median nerve function preoperatively and exploration of the nerve intraoperatively is expected. The carpal tunnel is routinely fully released in these injuries to facilitate both assessment and repair of injured structures. The order of repair in this zone is again deep to superficial, starting with the tendons then proceeding with exploration and repair of any nerve laceration.

In zone V, the myotendinous junction and muscle tissue are usually injured (**Fig. 10**). As there is less holding power of the suture in muscle tissue compared with tendon, locking sutures may be used to gain purchase in the thin tendinous material within the muscles. In cases of injury across flexors to multiple digits, each tendon must be carefully matched to the correct digit (**Fig. 11**). Importantly, the median nerve rests between the FDS and FDP tendon layers, which helps when defining the tendons. With careful tendon matching, a gentle cascade of increasing flexion from the index to small fingers should be restored.

PARTIAL TENDON LACERATIONS

Patients with partial tendon lacerations may still be able to flex the affected digit, but with pain or weakness. Historically, repair of partial tendon injuries was advocated due to concerns for bulbous scar tissue formation that could cause triggering and stiffness.[30] This was refuted by studies showing good clinical results without repairing partially injured tendons.[31,32] Biomechanical

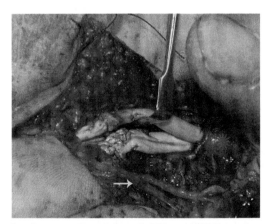

Fig. 9. Zone III repairs of FDS and FDP tendons showing greater room around tendons for repair proximal to A1 pulley (star). Note concomitant common digital nerve laceration which is common in this zone (*arrow*).

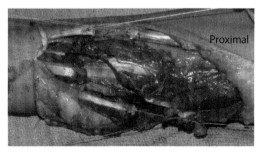

Fig. 10. Zone V laceration involving myotendinous structures with preparation for individual repairs using nonabsorbable suture placed in locking fashion on each end of lacerations.

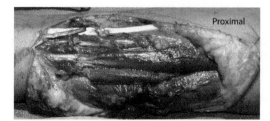

Fig. 11. Zone V laceration now with multiple tendons repaired. Repair sequence typically from deep to superficial.

studies have shown that tendon lacerations involving less than 60% of the tendon achieve superior results of higher load to failure and tensile strength with non-repair and early mobilization.[33,34] If half of a tendon remains intact, we would recommend debriding any cut edges to bevel them to a smooth surface and allowing unrestricted active motion afterwards (**Fig. 12**). We believe this is the most likely course of action to optimize motion of the injured and adjacent digits.

REHABILITATION

Over the past 50 years, there has been a tremendous evolution in rehabilitation of flexor tendon repair. In the early 1940s, Mason and Allen[4] showed in their study of canine extra-synovial tendon repairs that there was a 2 to 3 week period of obligate softening of the tendon ends and the diminution of the holding power of the suture. This led them to advocate for immobilization in the immediate postoperative period to decrease the risk of repair rupture.

As Mason and Allen's study, numerous studies have refuted the concern for repair site failure with early motion. In fact, early rehabilitation after flexor tendon repair has been recognized as key to promoting collagen deposition at the site of injury and preventing repair site rupture.

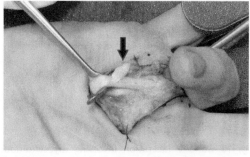

Fig. 12. Nonoperatively managed partial FDS laceration with flap of tendon (*arrow*) that was subsequently excised for symptomatic triggering.

Passive motion using rubber band traction immobilization was first described in 1960[35] and popularized in 1977 by the publication of the Louisville Protocol.[36] This described the use of a dorsal blocking plaster splint with rubber bands fixed to the fingers via a suture placed through the nail plate. This design allowed for active extension and passive flexion of the digits. The addition of a palmar bar was proposed in 1992 to redirect the force of pull more palmarly to increase PIP and DIP joint excursion.[37] Articulated splints allowing synergistic wrist motion have also been described.[38] The use of rubber bands, though, has been associated with flexion contractures and stiffness.[36]

In the modern era, rehabilitation programs are best described for zone II tendon injuries. There is a general acceptance that early mobilization starting within the first few postoperative days is desirable. Beyond that, there is no consensus program with surgeons and therapists pursuing a mix of active and passive motion protocols. One common protocol would use a dorsal blocking splint, with the wrist in 20 degrees of flexion, MP joints in 50 degrees of flexion, and extension at the IP joints. Passive flexion and extension exercises are used for the first 3 weeks, then transitioning to active motion within the splint is recommended. From the first therapy visit, some will modify this to include either place and hold flexion or mid-arc active flexion without resistance. The splint is removed for those active flexion and extension exercises. Splint wear at rest is typically maintained until 6 weeks postoperatively at which time most surgeons will allow unrestricted active motion without any resistance. Resistance exercises and strengthening are typically delayed until 12 weeks as flexor tendon repairs continue to accrue strength during that whole time.

Key biomechanical studies have guided these rehabilitation protocols. In a canine model, high excursion of the digit during rehabilitation did not prevent adhesion formation or improve tensile strength compared with low excursion exercises, suggesting that as little as 1.7 mm of excursion of the tendon is sufficient.[39] Furthermore, the amount of force applied across the repair site has not been shown to correlate with the accrual of tensile strength in repaired tendons.[18] These studies support the pursuit of early mobilization without the need for full range of motion or load.

We believe that the proper rehabilitation of flexor tendon injuries requires excellent communication. Surgeons must talk to the therapist to explain the quality of the tendon and the repair performed. The surgeon must also carefully explain the reason behind the prolonged restrictions and strict therapy to the patient so that the patient understands the importance of both doing the prescribed exercises and why they must be compliant with avoiding lifting or grabbing items. Similarly, therapists should be communicating with the surgeon about patient progress and individuals who may need to either be advanced or slowed in their program.

COMPLICATIONS

Despite intensive research in surgical techniques and rehabilitation, complications still occur after flexor tendon repair. Rupture at the repair site and adhesion formation remain the most common complications, each estimated to occur at a rate of 4%.[20] Age, gender, zone of injury, or rehabilitation method have not been found to predict complications.[20,40]

Adhesion formation occurs due to extrinsic healing and the ingrowth of external vascular supply. Extrinsic healing occurs via fibroblasts and inflammatory cells migrating to the repair site, whereas intrinsic healing relies on inflammatory cells within the tendon and epitenon.[15,41] Although tendon healing occurs by a combination of both intrinsic and extrinsic mechanisms, any predominance of extrinsic healing leads to scar buildup and adhesion formation. Early initiation of motion has been shown to be critical to preventing these intrasynovial adhesions.[39] On a cellular level, manipulating cytokine levels at the site of repair is an ongoing area of research.[42] If there is persistent lack of improvement in the range of active digital flexion, flexor tenolysis can be considered typically 3 to 6 months after repair. We recommend only performing a tenolysis when all progress with therapy has plateaued and soft tissues have reached an equilibrium signified by resolution of the initial firm, woody feel and the intermittent swelling that affects the injured digit for months.

Repair site rupture is a major complication, occurring at a rate of 4%. Possible contributing factors include core repair technique, not using a running epitendinous suture, and patient noncompliance with activity restriction. Treatment depends on the timing of the rupture and the amount of tendon end displacement. New advancements aimed at reducing the rate of repair site rupture include wide awake local anesthesia no tourniquet (WALANT) and intraoperative total active movement examination (iTAME), both aimed at assessing for any repair site gapping with active flexion intraoperatively.[43] If detected, this gapping can be repaired before leaving the operating room, as even a slight gap at time zero may be a harbinger for subsequent failure.

SUMMARY

Flexor tendon repair techniques and rehabilitation have advanced tremendously in the past 50 years. However, the attributes of the ideal tendon repair articulated by Dr Strickland in 1995 hold true today.[44] The ideal repair requires sutures easily placed in the tendon, secure suture knots, a smooth juncture of tendon ends, minimal gapping, minimal interference with tendon vascularity, and sufficient strength throughout healing. When accomplished, the modern flexor tendon repair is a stout repair, sufficient for early mobilization and intrinsic tendon healing.

CLINICS CARE POINTS

- Flexor tendon repairs require both precise repairs and dedication to rehabilitation to achieve optimal results
- For active motion rehabilitation, flexor tendon repairs require a minimum of four core suture strands
- Following flexor tendon repair, gapping must remain under 3 mm for the tendon to accrue normal strength
- In zone II repairs, visualization of the distal tendon stump through the pulley system should guide judicious placement of pulley releases necessary for repairs

DISCLOSURE

No disclosures with commercial companies for either author.

REFERENCES

1. Kleinert HE, Spokevicius S, Papas NH. History of flexor tendon repair. J Hand Surg Am 1995;20(3 Pt 2):S46–52.
2. Bunnell S. Repair of tendons in the fingers and description of two new instruments. Surg Gynecol Obstet 1918;26:103–10.
3. Bunnell S. Repair of tendons in the fingers. Surg Gynecol Obstet 1922;35:88–97.
4. Mason ML, Allen HS. The rate of healing of tendons: an experimental study of tensile strength. Ann Surg 1941;113(3):424–59.
5. Gelberman RH, Vande Berg JS, Lundborg GN, et al. Flexor tendon healing and restoration of the gliding surface. An ultrastructural study in dogs. J Bone Joint Surg Am 1983;65(1):70–80.

6. Gelberman RH, Nunley JA 2nd, Osterman AL, et al. Influences of the protected passive mobilization interval on flexor tendon healing. A prospective randomized clinical study. Clin Orthop Relat Res 1991;(264):189–96.

7. Lundborg G. Experimental flexor tendon healing without adhesion formation–a new concept of tendon nutrition and intrinsic healing mechanisms. A preliminary report. Hand 1976;8(3):235–8.

8. Trumble TE, Vedder NB, Benirschke SK. Misleading fractures after profundus tendon avulsions: a report of six cases. J Hand Surg Am 1992;17(5):902–6.

9. Al-Qattan MM. Type 5 avulsion of the insertion of the flexor digitorum profundus tendon. J Hand Surg Br 2001;26(5):427–31.

10. McCallister WV, Ambrose HC, Katolik LI, et al. Comparison of pullout button versus suture anchor for zone I flexor tendon repair. J Hand Surg Am 2006; 31(2):246–51.

11. Compton J, Wall LB, Romans S, et al. Outcomes of acute repair versus nonrepair of zone I Flexor digitorum profundus tendon injuries. J Hand Surg Am 2022. https://doi.org/10.1016/j.jhsa.2022.02.005. S0363-5023(22)00120-4. Online ahead of print.

12. de Jong JP, Nguyen JT, Sonnema AJ, et al. The incidence of acute traumatic tendon injuries in the hand and wrist: a 10-year population-based study. Clin Orthop Surg 2014;6(2):196–202.

13. Gelberman RH, Boyer MI, Brodt MD, et al. The effect of gap formation at the repair site on the strength and excursion of intrasynovial flexor tendons. An experimental study on the early stages of tendon-healing in dogs. J Bone Joint Surg Am 1999;81(7): 975–82.

14. Manske PR, Gelberman RH, Vande Berg JS, et al. Intrinsic flexor-tendon repair. A morphological study in vitro. J Bone Joint Surg Am 1984;66(3):385–96.

15. Lundborg G, Rank F. Experimental intrinsic healing of flexor tendons based upon synovial fluid nutrition. J Hand Surg Am 1978;3(1):21–31.

16. Zhao C, Amadio PC, Paillard P, et al. Digital resistance and tendon strength during the first week after flexor digitorum profundus tendon repair in a canine model in vivo. J Bone Joint Surg Am 2004;86(2):320–7.

17. Osei DA, Stepan JG, Calfee RP, et al. The effect of suture caliber and number of core suture strands on zone II flexor tendon repair: a study in human cadavers. J Hand Surg Am 2014;39(2):262–8.

18. Boyer MI, Gelberman RH, Burns ME, et al. Intrasynovial flexor tendon repair. An experimental study comparing low and high levels of in vivo force during rehabilitation in canines. J Bone Joint Surg Am 2001; 83(6):891–9.

19. Taras JS, Raphael JS, Marczyk SC, et al. Evaluation of suture caliber in flexor tendon repair. J Hand Surg Am 2001;26(6):1100–4.

20. Dy CJ, Hernandez-Soria A, Ma Y, et al. Complications after flexor tendon repair: a systematic review and meta-analysis. J Hand Surg Am 2012;37(3): 543–551 e541.

21. Diao E, Hariharan JS, Soejima O, et al. Effect of peripheral suture depth on strength of tendon repairs. J Hand Surg Am 1996;21(2):234–9.

22. Dinopoulos HT, Boyer MI, Burns ME, et al. The resistance of a four- and eight-strand suture technique to gap formation during tensile testing: an experimental study of repaired canine flexor tendons after 10 days of in vivo healing. J Hand Surg Am 2000; 25(3):489–98.

23. Tang JB, Zhang Y, Cao Y, et al. Core suture purchase affects strength of tendon repairs. J Hand Surg Am 2005;30(6):1262–6.

24. Bunnell S. Surgery of the hand. Surgery of the hand, Lippincott. Jb 1944;298.

25. Tang JB. Indications, methods, postoperative motion and outcome evaluation of primary flexor tendon repairs in Zone 2. J Hand Surg Eur 2007;32(2): 118–29.

26. Mitsionis G, Bastidas JA, Grewal R, et al. Feasibility of partial A2 and A4 pulley excision: effect on finger flexor tendon biomechanics. J Hand Surg Am 1999; 24(2):310–4.

27. Savage R. The mechanical effect of partial resection of the digital fibrous flexor sheath. J Hand Surg Br 1990;15(4):435–42.

28. Tang J, Shi D, Gu Y. [Flexor tendon repair: timing of surgery and sheath management]. Zhonghua Wai Ke Za Zhi 1995;33(9):532–5.

29. Al-Qattan MM. Flexor tendon repair in zone III. J Hand Surg Eur 2011;36(1):48–52.

30. Schlenker JD, Lister GD, Kleinert HE. Three complications of untreated partial laceration of flexor tendon–entrapment, rupture, and triggering. J Hand Surg Am 1981;6(4):392–8.

31. Wray RC Jr, Holtman B, Weeks PM. Clinical treatment of partial tendon lacerations without suturing and with early motion. Plast Reconstr Surg 1977; 59(2):231–4.

32. McGeorge DD, Stilwell JH. Partial flexor tendon injuries: to repair or not. J Hand Surg Br 1992;17(2): 176–7.

33. Bishop AT, Cooney WP 3rd, Wood MB. Treatment of partial flexor tendon lacerations: the effect of tenorrhaphy and early protected mobilization. J Trauma 1986;26(4):301–12.

34. Ollinger H, Wray RC Jr, Weeks PM. Effects of suture on tensile strength gain of partially and completely severed tendons. Surg Forum 1975;26:63–4.

35. Hitchcock TF, Light TR, Bunch WH, et al. The effect of immediate constrained digital motion on the strength of flexor tendon repairs in chickens. J Hand Surg Am 1987;12(4):590–5.

36. Lister GD, Kleinert HE, Kutz JE, et al. Primary flexor tendon repair followed by immediate controlled mobilization. J Hand Surg Am 1977;2(6):441–51.

37. Horii E, Lin GT, Cooney WP, et al. Comparative flexor tendon excursion after passive mobilization: an in vitro study. J Hand Surg Am 1992;17(3):559–66.

38. Chow JA, Thomes LJ, Dovelle S, et al. A combined regimen of controlled motion following flexor tendon repair in "no man's land". Plast Reconstr Surg 1987; 79(3):447–55.

39. Silva MJ, Brodt MD, Boyer MI, et al. Effects of increased in vivo excursion on digital range of motion and tendon strength following flexor tendon repair. J Orthop Res 1999;17(5):777–83.

40. Chesney A, Chauhan A, Kattan A, et al. Systematic review of flexor tendon rehabilitation protocols in zone II of the hand. Plast Reconstr Surg 2011; 127(4):1583–92.

41. Manske PR, Lesker PA. Flexor tendon nutrition. Hand Clin 1985;1(1):13–24.

42. Beredjiklian PK. Biologic aspects of flexor tendon laceration and repair. J Bone Joint Surg Am 2003; 85(3):539–50.

43. Higgins A, Lalonde DH, Bell M, et al. Avoiding flexor tendon repair rupture with intraoperative total active movement examination. Plast Reconstr Surg 2010; 126(3):941–5.

44. Strickland JW. Flexor Tendon Injuries: II. Operative Technique. J Am Acad Orthop Surg 1995;3(1):55–62.

Flexor Tendon Repair Techniques: M-Tang Repair

Jin Bo Tang, MD[a],*, Zhang Jun Pan, MD[b], Giovanni Munz, MD[c,d], Inga S. Besmens, MD[e], Leila Harhaus, MD[f,g]

KEYWORDS

- Flexor tendon repair • M-Tang techniques • Peripheral suture • Pulley venting • Early active flexion
- Outcomes

KEY POINTS

- Primary or delayed primary repair of digital flexor tendons are both feasible. The timing of surgery is not important if the repair is not delayed too long (eg, 5 weeks).
- The lacerated tendon is approached through a 2 to 3 cm incision. If the proximal tendon stumps are retracted, an incision in the distal palm is made to find them.
- The M-Tang six-strand core repair is made with two groups of 4-0 looped nylon forming an M shape in the tendon. The suture purchase should be 0.7 to 1 cm in each tendon stump, and the repair should be placed under some tension to prevent gapping.
- The peripheral suture can be a sparse circle or cross sutures with 5-0 suture or running sutures with 6-0 nylon. Some surgeons do not use peripheral suture after six-strand M-Tang repair.
- The pulley should be vented if needed, and postoperative early active flexion exercise starts from 4 to 5 days after surgery with the active flexion to half or 2/3 of the digital flexion arc.

INTRODUCTION

We have repaired lacerated flexor tendons within 4 to 5 weeks and have found similar outcomes with primary repairs immediately after surgery. With a strong repair technique, early active flexion is possible in patients whose flexor tendons are repaired after weeks of delay, with minimal risk for rupture.

SURGICAL METHODS
Surgical Incisions

The lacerated flexor tendons in the finger are approached through the laceration and a volar distal extension for 2 to 3 cm, just enough to expose the tendons and carry out the repair.[1]

The small incision of 2 to 3 cm diminishes edema in the finger and resistance to tendon gliding during early active flexion exercise after surgery (**Figs. 1** and **2**). An extension of the incision is usually in the skin distal to the laceration (see **Fig. 1**), because the finger is commonly cut in digital flexion and the distal tendon end lies distal to the site of laceration. Proximal extension of the incision is sometimes needed. However, a lengthy proximal extension is not recommended.

Instead, a separate 1 cm incision is made in the distal palm to find the stump of the flexor digitorum profundus (FDP), which is delivered to the repair site in the finger (**Fig. 3**A, B). The FDP tendon is found beneath the flexor digitorum superficialis (FDS) tendon and is grasped with two sets of

[a] Department of Hand Surgery, The Hand Surgery Research Center, Affiliated Hospital of Nantong University, Nantong, Jiangsu, China; [b] Hand Surgery, Yixing City Hospital, Yixing, Jiangsu, China; [c] Azienda Ospedaliera Careggi: Azienda Ospedaliero Universitaria Careggi, Surgery and microsurgery of the hand, Largo Palagi 1, Firenze, Italy; [d] Current position is: Unit of hand surgery, Santo Stefano Hospital, via Suor Niccolina Infermiera 22, Prato, Italy; [e] Department of Plastic Surgery and Hand Surgery, University Hospital Zurich, Switzerland; [f] Department of Hand, Plastic and Reconstructive Surgery, Burn Center, BG Trauma Center Ludwigshafen, Heidelberg, Germany; [g] Department of Hand and Plastic Surgery, University of Heidelberg, Heidelberg, Germany
* Corresponding author.
E-mail address: jinbotang@yahoo.com

Hand Clin 39 (2023) 141–149
https://doi.org/10.1016/j.hcl.2022.08.015

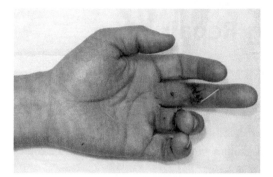

Fig. 1. Clinical photo of a patient who sustained lacerations to the left long, ring, and small fingers. Planned extension distally of the long finger laceration to a total of 2 cm is depicted by the yellow line. **Figs. 1–3** and **8** are from the same patient. (*Courtesy of* Jin Bo Tang, MD, Jiangsu, China.)

forceps (see **Fig. 3**A). The tendon is pushed distally with the proximal forceps with the distal ones released, and the distal forceps are then moved proximally to grasp and push again. Repeating the maneuver a few times can advance the proximal stump into the surgical incision in the finger (see **Fig. 3**B).

Making a Core Suture

We use a six-strand M-Tang repair (**Fig. 4**).[2–5] A four-strand repair meets basic requirements regarding repair strength. We observed that after completion of a four-strand repair, the repair site usually has remarkable pliability and gaps on stretching; however, after placing two additional strands, the repair site shows much greater firmness and resistance to gapping when pulled. We always perform a six-strand repair in zone 2. Eight or more strands are reasonable but are used by fewer surgeons or in special cases requiring a more robust repair.[6]

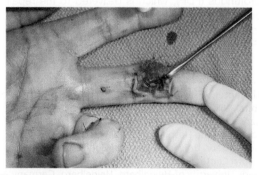

Fig. 2. Venting of the entire A4 for exposure and tendon repair. The FDP tendon was lacerated at the border of zone 2A and zone 1. (*Courtesy of* Jin Bo Tang, MD, Jiangsu, China.)

In placing the core suture, it is critical to keep its purchase of at least 7 to 10 mm in each tendon stump.[5,7,8] There are four locks in the M-Tang repair. The lock size should be 2 mm in diameter when a locking suture is used. A 4-0 or 3-0 looped nonabsorbable nonbraided suture is used. A 4-0 looped monofilament nylon such as Supramid Extra (S. Jackson, Inc., Alexandria, VA) is used in tendons in the digit area of my patients (JBT). We do not favor Ethibond (Ethicon, Inc., Somerville, NJ) suture in zone 2 repair because it is hard to keep under tension and easily becomes loose. We prefer a needle of a larger size but have no particular preference regarding needle types. In making the M-Tang repair, we first finish a U-shaped repair with one looped suture, then 2 strands are added to the center of the tendon with another looped suture (**Figure 4**). In our repairs with an M-Tang method, knots are exposed on the tendon surface, mostly on the lateral and volar aspects of the tendon.

The core suture should be six-strand and tensioned to make the junction site slightly bulky. The allowed bulkiness ranges from 20% to 30%, up to 50% increase in the diameter of the repaired tendon (**Fig. 5**).

Peripheral Suture

The core suture should be six-strand and tensioned to make the junction site slightly bulky. The allowed bulkiness ranges from 20% to 30%, up to 50% increase in the diameter of the repaired tendon (**Fig. 5**).

We believe that a strong six-strand core suture does not require a peripheral suture, but adding a few sutures may help further reduce gliding resistance in early active flexion of the operated digits (**Fig. 6**A–E). Performing a *digital extension-flexion test* is a must after any peripheral suture or when the surgeon decides not to add peripheral suture, as this test shows whether the junction site need additional tightening with a few peripheral sutures (**Fig. 7**).

JUDICIOUS VENTING OF ANNULAR PULLEYS

Although it was not acceptable 20 years ago, pulley venting is now considered critical to ensure functional recovery and is unlikely to cause clinical problems when executed cautiously.[9–17] Narrow and rigid annular pulleys restrict tendon gliding and block motion of the edematous tendon repair site. Therefore, release of these pulleys (or their most narrow parts) improves tendon motion, thereby decreasing the risk of rupture during early active digital motion.[9–16] Nevertheless, such releases should be executed

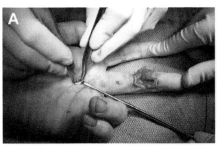
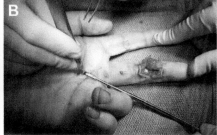

Fig. 3. Delivery of the retracted FDP tendon by making a separate small incision in the palm. (*A*) Two sets of forceps were used to grasp the tendon in the palm through an incision in the distal palm. (*B*) The proximal forceps pushed the FDP tendon to the incision in the finger distally. (*Courtesy of* Jin Bo Tang, MD, Jiangsu, China.)

cautiously to avoid creating a lengthy sheath-pulley defect and damaging the series of annular pulleys. A sheath-pulley release less than 2 cm long causes no clinical tendon bowstringing, provided that other portions of the sheath and pulleys are preserved. A slightly wider venting such as venting the A4 with A3 is also allowable when necessary.[3,10,11]

Two essential rules are as follows: (1) a segment of the A2 pulley should always be retained (the venting can be distal or proximal to the retained A2 portion, which may include the entire A1 pulley or cruciate pulleys distal to the A2 pulley) and (2) the A4 pulley can be entirely vented, including extension to the A3 pulley, but should not extend over or much proximal to the A3 pulley. Occasionally, the A2 pulley will have to be entirely vented, but this is not customary.

Retaining at least a part—up to one-half or two-thirds of the A2 pulley—is a safe recommendation for venting.[2,5]

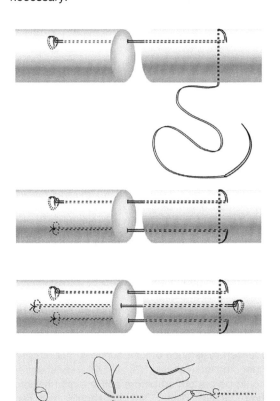

Fig. 4. Making a six-strand M-Tang repair with two groups of looped sutures. The yellow penal shows how to make a start lock (left) and end lock (middle and right). (*From* Tang JB, Zhou X, Pan ZJ, et al. Strong digital flexor tendon repair, extension-flexion test, and early active flexion: experience in 300 tendons. Hand Clin. 2017, 33:455–63; with permission.)

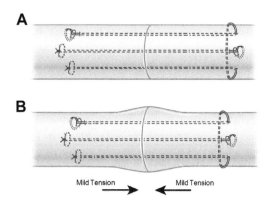

Mild Tension →   ← Mild Tension

Fig. 5. Ensuring sufficient tension across the repair is a key to surgical repair. (*A*) A very flat repair easily develops gapping when the tendon is pulled proximally during early active digital flexion. (*B*) Slightly bulkiness at the junction site is preferred and the junction site would be flatter when being pulled proximally during active flexion exercise. Mild bulkiness at repair site is not a major problem to tendon gliding with proper pulley-venting. An increase in the repair site diameter by one-fifth to one-fourth is tolerable after completion of the repair, before removal of the temporary fixation needle to the proximal tendon stump. However, remarkable bulkiness at the repair site should always be avoided. (*From* Tang JB, Zhou X, Pan ZJ, et al. Strong digital flexor tendon repair, extension-flexion test, and early active flexion: experience in 300 tendons. Hand Clin. 2017, 33:455–63; with permission.)

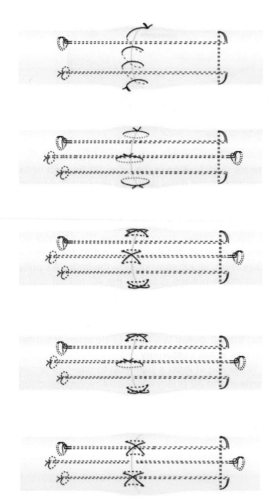

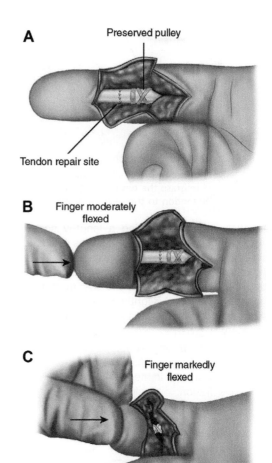

Fig. 6. Several simpler peripheral sutures with a strong six-strand core suture repair; 5 to 0 or 6 to 0 sutures are used for a few different types of simpler peripheral sutures. (*Adapted from* Pan ZJ, Xu YF, Pan L, Chen J. Zone 2 flexor tendon repairs using a tensioned strong core suture, sparse peripheral stitches and early active motion: results in 60 fingers. J Hand Surg Eur Vol. 2019;44(4):361-66. with permission.)

Fig. 7. The digital extension–flexion test has three parts: (*A*) full extension; (*B*) moving from full extension to moderate flexion; and (*C*) moving toward full flexion. (*From* Tang JB, Zhou X, Pan ZJ, et al. Strong digital flexor tendon repair, extension-flexion test, and early active flexion: experience in 300 tendons. Hand Clin. 2017, 33:455–63; with permission)

COMBINED PASSIVE–ACTIVE MOTION WITH A SHORTER SPLINT

Increasingly, much shorter splints are used for protection of the wrist and hand after flexor tendon repair.[18,19] A short splint extends from either the distal forearm or the wrist to the fingertips. Most of us use a splint from the distal forearm to the fingertips. In addition, wrist positions can be varied. The wrist can be in neutral, mild flexion, or mild extension, provided that the patient is comfortable. The splint should be slightly flexed at the metacarpophalangeal joint and be straight beyond the metacarpophalangeal joint, should extend past the finger or thumb tip, and should avoid marked flexion or extension.

Therapy is begun from day 4 or 5, with at least a few sessions of digital motion exercises daily; the exact number of sessions should be decided by the surgeon and therapist according to preferences and the patient's condition. In each session, to lessen resistance of joint stiffness, full passive finger motion—usually 20 to 40 repetitions—should be performed before active digital flexion. Then, active digital flexion should proceed gradually.

More recently, the lead author proposes an increase in the number of runs to a minimal of 40 runs of active flexion in each session in home-based exercise, and there should be 4 to 6 sessions of motion exercise each day at home, so the patient can be ensured with sufficient motion runs in each session.[20]

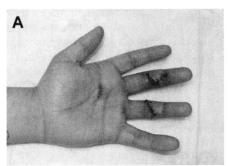 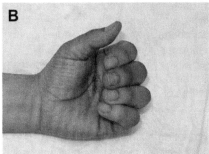

Fig. 8. Out-of-splint motion in the first 3 to 4 weeks after repair of the same patient with very mild edema in the finger. (*A*) Full extension of the finger and (*B*) partial range active flexion. (*Courtesy of* Jin Bo Tang, MD, Jiangsu, China)

In the first 3 to 4 weeks, only one-third to two-thirds of the active motion range should be the goal (**Fig. 8**A, B). Extreme digital active flexion should be avoided, because the tendon has greatly increased resistance to gliding and the repair is more prone to rupture when the tendon is bent and pulled.[2,3,20] In reality, some patients have marked swelling at this time, making full range of active motion difficult. For these patients, it is not possible to immediately pursue forceful, full active flexion, but full passive finger flexion and extension should always be performed.

From the end of week 3 or 4, full range of active flexion is the goal. Patients having difficulty with full active flexion at week 4 or 5 may gradually achieve full flexion in later weeks, but exercise to reduce joint stiffness and prevent extension lag is very important for eventual recovery of active finger flexion.

Out-of-splint active motion is encouraged as the most efficient exercise for decreasing resistance to active motion (see **Fig. 8**A, B). A robust tendon repair is strong enough to permit the digit to move out of splint. The splint can be discarded entirely at week 6 to 7 depending on the severity of injury. Rehabilitation should continue for at least 8 to 10 weeks postoperatively (or longer), with the goal of decreasing residual extension lag or achieving full flexion. After flexor pollicis longus (FPL) repairs, active thumb flexion exercise is similar to that of the fingers, although some details vary.[21,22]

Variants of Treatment Methods and Outcomes Documented from Different Institutes

Here, we present the variants of methods and outcomes documented or reported from the different institutes of the authors.

Nantong University, Nantong
Between January 2017 and January 2020, 81 fingers in 73 consecutive patients with complete divisions of the FDP tendon were treated.[23] At the time of final follow-up, nine patients could not be traced due to changes in addresses or phone numbers, and 31 patients refused to come to the hospital for follow-up. We reviewed 37 fingers (12 index, 7 middle, 9 ring, and 9 little) in 33 patients (10 women and 23 men) with a mean age of 37 years (range 19–70). Three fingers had the FDP tendon injured in zone 1, 31 in zone 2, and three in zone 3. The patients were followed for a mean of 19 months (range 8–39) postoperatively. There were no repair ruptures, and no fingers needed tenolysis.[23] The results are graded according to the Tang criteria in 31 fingers injured in zone 2. Excellent and good results were found in 26 fingers (84%), whereas we had three fair and two poor outcomes.[23] This is the most recent audit of the patients. In earlier years, the outcomes were similar. The excellent and good rates were around 85% with no ruptures and only a very few digits in need of tenolysis. In the most recent 3 years, we had no fingers that needed tenolysis.

We noted over years there have been some unfortunate patients, with about 10% to 15% of the fingers not reaching good outcomes, mainly because joint stiffness or multiple finger involvement. The patients with fractures or soft tissue defects are not included into the audits as these patients have other major structural damages, which affect outcomes more than flexor tendon injuries themselves.

Yixing City Hospital, Yixing
The methods used and outcomes have been detailed in recent reports.[24,25] We performed regular audits in all of our patients with zone 2 repair in the fingers and thumbs after we implemented updated methods and motion protocols over the past 8 years.[24] We only had ruptures of three FDP tendons in fingers out of more than 200 fingers and thumbs with zone 2 FDP or FPL repair, no rupture in the patients who did out-of-splint

early active motion and no rupture in FPL tendons. We typically use sparsely located separate stitches of peripheral suture with 5-0 suture using nylon or prolene, as this is fast and strong.[24,25] We do not repair the FDS tendon except a partial FDS cut, and the constricting pulleys are vented with a length limit of 2 cm. The early motion exercise (Nantong protocol) starts from day 4 to 6 after surgery.

The patients with finger stiffness improve over months, and follow-up after a year usually reveals good finger motion even if these fingers are graded as fair initially. Therefore, there is no rush for tenolysis for the mild cases.

The setting can be simple, but the keys are *surgeon's mastery of surgical techniques and adherence to all needed principles*. A strong repair method must be used and an extension–flexion test is performed, followed by true active flexion exercise after surgery (with or without therapists' involvement). The surgeons should understand *all* these key considerations should be met, and senior surgeons need to teach the junior colleagues to adhere to *all, not part*, of these requirements. With these key steps involving reading updated texts and watching surgical videos, we changed from an incidence of 20% ruptures of the zone 2 repair before 2014 to 0% rupture in zone 2 of those who followed instructions starting in 2014. Over the past 8 years from 2014, rupture occurred in three FDP tendons (1.2%) of zone 2 in the first a few weeks after surgery in those who forcefully used their hands.[24,25]

Azienda Ospedaliero Universitaria Careggi, Florence

Dr Munz and his colleagues carried out delayed primary repair of flexor tendons in zone 2 in 31 fingers and thumb (28 patients) averaging 15 days (range 4–37) after injury in 2020 in this institute.[4] The delay was longer than usual due to the COVID-19 pandemic. The tendons were repaired with a six-strand M-Tang method or a double-Tsuge suture and a simple running peripheral suture or sparse peripheral stitches. This was followed by an early, partial-range, active flexion exercise program. Adhesions in four digits required tenolysis.[4] These patients who had tenolysis were not those who presented with longest delay. Outcomes of two improved after tenolysis. The other two patients declined further surgery, and improvement was noted. One finger flexor tendon ruptured in early active motion. This was re-repaired, and final outcome was good. Overall excellent and good results using the Tang criteria were in 27 of 31 fingers and thumbs (87%).[4] The time elapsed between the injury and

surgery is not an important risk factor for a good outcome, rather it depends on proper surgical methods, the surgeon's experience, and early mobilization, properly applied. Munz and colleagues found adhesions may occur in a small percent of the patients, but they can be managed with tenolysis.[4]

University of Zurich, Zurich

We believe that a main predictor for a good outcome in flexor tendon repair is to perform a strong core suture repair that will allow for a controlled active motion rehabilitation protocol.[26] We do not usually add peripheral suture after a repair six-strand M-Tang repair. We found division of the A3 pulley together with the A4 do not cause clinically significant functional disturbance. Therefore, we divide two pulleys together if necessary. With these considerations in mind, we have reached favorable outcomes after primary or delayed tendon repair over the last decade.

Between January 2014 and December 2016, 29 patients (32 digits, including 5 thumbs and 27 fingers) with complete divisions of the FDP tendon in zone 1C or zone 2 (27 fingers) and FPL tendon in zone 2 (5 thumbs) were treated by primary or delayed primary repair.[3] We did not add a circumferential repair after a six-strand M-Tang repair. The outcomes of the 27 fingers were excellent in 18, good in 6, fair in 2, and poor in 1. There was no repair rupture in the first 3 years. Between 2017 and 2021, we repaired (and have a full postoperative data set for) 84 flexor tendons (18 FPL and 66 FDP) in zones 1 to 3 in 80 patients with the above mentioned technique in our department. The mean time between injury and surgery was 3 days (0–39 days). The 66 FDP tendon repairs included 27 in the index finger, 12 in the middle finger, 7 in the ring finger, and 20 in the little finger. We registered tendon ruptures in six patients (6 digits): three of those repairs were performed in zone 1, two in zone 2, and one in zone 3. Two ruptures were registered for FPL tendons: two in the index finger and two in the little finger. Of the six patients, only four wished to undergo revision surgery, that is, immediate re-repair. We found no explanation for the ruptures that we encountered, but it may relate to the learning curve of new surgeons. As we are working in a teaching institution, the level of experience of the operating surgeons varies greatly, though of course a senior surgeon always supervises the surgeries. Such ruptures may relate to less supervised exercises after surgery during the pandemic.

Although functional outcomes were not fully audited in the recent 4 years, functional outcomes were generally similar to what we reported in 2018[3], and secondary tenolysis is infrequently needed. Therefore, the surgical techniques and postoperative therapy that we currently used are the same with those used between 2014 and 2017 and reported earlier.[3,27–30] Regarding suture materials, we now regularly use Supramid (4-0, DRT 18mm needle, RESORBA Medical GmbH, Nürnberg, Germany) to make the 6-strand M-Tang repair. We use a circumferential running suture in very few circumstances, typically where the tendon stumps are irregular or there is a risk of repair snagging.

Heidelberg University, Heidelberg

One challenge for us is how to introduce new surgical and therapeutic concepts into departments that have used traditional techniques for decades. Using the knowledge of novel learning theories, we undertook changing our traditional Kirchmayr–Kessler tendon suture and postoperative Washington motion protocol to the new M-Tang repair method and Manchester motion protocol in our department of about 40 hand surgeons and 40 physio- and occupational therapists beginning in 2020. The aim was to standardize the suture technique and motion protocols and to maintain the clinical standards over time and included step-by-step videos which were prepared and published in *our in-house App* (**Fig. 9**). We established

a training station where every surgeon had to perform the new suture technique under documented supervision of the experts.[1]

A recheck of surgeons' performance was performed after 6 months as a quality control, when each surgeon had to demonstrate the technique again at this working station. Following the surgeons' quality checks, we started the change process for the postoperative motion protocol. For further quality control, we followed our patients after 3, 6, and 12 weeks and assessed all details including wound condition, edema, active range of digital motion, and patients' reports on their experiences with the Manchester protocol of the early active motion.

From January 2020 to December 2021, we performed 408 flexor tendon repairs in zone 2 using the new suture technique and the new postoperative motion protocol as described above. There were 408 digits (61 thumbs and 347 fingers). The suture materials for making the M-Tang repair was Fiberloop 4-0 (Arthrex, Munich, Germany). We added a peritendinous suture using 5-0 polydioxanone (Ethicon, Norderstedt, Germany). The pulleys were vented as needed, and the FDS repaired only when it did not affect the FDP gliding capacity. Out of these, we had 13 ruptures (rupture incidence 3.2%), which happened mostly during "too motivated exercises" for these patients. In revision surgery, seven digits received secondary

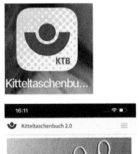
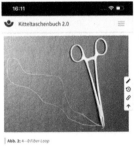
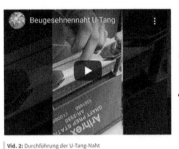
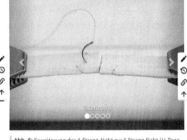

Deliberate training of surgical techniques of M-Tang repair in Heideberg University, Germany, with an intra-departmental app is shown. The training bypassed clinical learning curves and ensured universal improvement in outcomes of flexor tendon repairs in zone 2 in 2020-2021 in 408 digits (61 thumbs and 347 fingers) with few ruptures and few tenolysis.

Fig. 9. Flowchart of training of the M-Tang tendon repair method used in Heidelberg, Germany. Extracts of the dedicated chapter on M-Tang tendon repair in the in-house knowledge-App of Heidelberg, Germany.

M-Tang sutures, three digits received tendon grafts when the quality of the ruptured tendon was too poor for secondary direct repair, and three digits underwent two-stage reconstruction and then healed uneventfully.

Dalhousie University, Saint John, Canada

Dr Donald Lalonde in Saint John, Canada, published his currently used methods and technical keys as follows[1]: Make short incisions with a separate incision in the palm if needed to decrease adhesions and the need for tenolysis. Push the palm tendons distally with two forceps so the FDP stays inside the FDS decussation. Grab the cut tendon ends as little as possible because you should not injure the cells you are asking to heal.

To decrease tenolysis incidence to almost zero, make sure you vent enough pulley that a slightly bunched, very sturdy repair does not impair full-fist active flexion and full extension testing in the awake patient. Vent either A2 or A4 as required, but avoid clinically obvious bowstringing by venting no more than a total of 1.5 to 2 cm of pulley.[11,26] Small amounts of bowstringing demonstrated in wide-awake surgery with active full-fist flexion and extension testing are well tolerated and not clinically important.

To decrease rupture incidence to almost zero, make very solid six-strand M-Tang repairs (4-0, Supramid, S. Jackson, VA) with 1-cm bites. Test all repairs with active full-fist flexion and extension in a wide-awake setting. Patients need to look at their hand to be able to know where their numb fingers are in space. If you see a gap form with testing, do not leave it as it will lead to rupture. To repair a gap: (1) do not remove the first loose suture as this is unnecessary tendon trauma that will lead to more scarring and decreased tendon blood supply; (2) insert a second tighter suture but leave the ends long when you tie the knot of the second suture; (3) tighten the first loose suture by pulling on one of its loops or its knot until it is as tight as it should be; and (4) take the loose loop or knot of the first tightened suture and tie it to the long ends of the second suture.

A partial range active flexion exercise program is used from day 4 or 5. In none of the patients, place and hold is used. In the later period of therapy, relative motion splint is used for those patients who are found to have adhesions. Dr Lalonde has had almost zero rupture of the repair in recent years, and few patients needed tenolysis.[31]

SUMMARY

The outcomes from six institutes with M-Tang repair with early active postoperative flexion are none or close to none repair rupture and very few digits needing tenolysis. The excellent and good rate is generally between 80% and 90%. In the pandemic period, less stringent therapy supervision might have allowed some patients move too aggressively, with repair ruptures not seen before the pandemic in one institute. In Nantong, Yixing, and Saint John, the rupture incidence is zero to about 1%. In Florence and Heidelberg, the rupture incidence was 3%, and the patients needing secondary reconstruction was less than 1%. In Zurich, the rupture incidence was zero from 2014 to 2017, but in recent audits several ruptures were found, which might have been caused by irregular visits to therapists and less stringent supervision of therapy during pandemic. Two institutes had an extremely large number of patients (>200 repairs) treated with the M-Tang repair technique, and their postoperative therapy regimens are very similar. In the two institutes—one from Asia and the other from Europe—there were always some patients who did not follow instructions of surgeons or therapists. The ruptures of the repair in these patients are beyond the control of surgeons or therapists.

CLINICS CARE POINTS

- Primary or delayed primary repair of digital flexor tendons are both feasible. The lacerated tendon is approached through a small incision of 2 to 3 cm. If proximal tendon stumps are retracted, an incision in the distal palm is made to find the tendon ends.

- M-Tang six-strand core repair is made with two groups of 4 to 0 looped nylon forming an M shape in the tendon. The suture purchase should be 0.7 to 1 cm in each tendon stump, and repair should have some tension to prevent gapping.

- Peripheral suture can be sparse circle or cross sutures with 5-0 suture, or running sutures with 6-0 nylon. Some surgeons do not use peripheral suture after 6-strand M-Tang repair.

- The restrictive pulley should be vented if needed, but the length of such venting should be less than 1.5 to 2 cm. Postoperative early active flexion exercise starts from 4 to 5 days after surgery with the active flexion to half or 2/3 of the digital flexion arc. In the later therapy period, relative motion splint is very helpful to correct tendon adhesions.

- Deliberate training of surgical repair techniques is recommended to bypass clinical learning curve.

REFERENCES

1. Tang JB, Lalonde D, Harhaus L, et al. Flexor tendon repair: recent changes and current methods. J Hand Surg Eur 2022;47:31–9.

2. Tang JB. Flexor tendon injuries. Clin Plast Surg 2019;46:295–306.

3. Giesen T, Reissner L, Besmens I, et al. Flexor tendon repair in the hand with the M-Tang technique (without peripheral sutures), pulley division, and early active motion. J Hand Surg Eur 2018;43:474–9.

4. Munz G, Poggetti A, Cenci L, et al. Up to five-week delay in primary repair of Zone 2 flexor tendon injuries: outcomes and complications. J Hand Surg Eur 2021;46:818–24.

5. Tang JB. Indications, methods, postoperative motion and outcome evaluation of primary flexor tendon repairs in zone. J Hand Surg Eur 2007;32:118–29.

6. Tang JB. Uncommon methods of flexor tendon and tendon-bone repairs and grafting. Hand Clin 2013; 29:215–21.

7. Cao Y, Zhu B, Xie RG, et al. Influence of core suture purchase length on strength of four-strand tendon repairs. J Hand Surg Am 2006;31:107–12.

8. Tang JB, Zhang Y, Cao Y, et al. Core suture purchase affects strength of tendon repairs. J Hand Surg Am 2005;30:1262–6.

9. Tang JB. New developments are improving flexor tendon repair. Plast Reconstr Surg 2018;141: 1427–37.

10. Tang JB. Recent evolutions in flexor tendon repairs and rehabilitation. J Hand Surg Eur 2018;43:469–73.

11. Tang JB, Zhou X, Pan ZJ, et al. Strong digital flexor tendon repair, extension-flexion test, and early active flexion: experience in 300 tendons. Hand Clin 2017;33:455–63.

12. Kwai Ben I, Elliot D. Venting" or partial lateral release of the A2 and A4 pulleys after repair of zone 2 flexor tendon injuries. J Hand Surg Br 1998;23:649–54.

13. Elliot D, Giesen T. Primary flexor tendon surgery: The search for a perfect result. Hand Clin 2013;29: 191–206.

14. Tang JB. Release of the A4 pulley to facilitate zone II flexor tendon repair. J Hand Surg Am 2014;39: 2300–7.

15. Tang JB, Chang J, Elliot D, et al. IFSSH Flexor Tendon Committee report 2014: From the IFSSH Flexor Tendon Committee (Chairman: Jin Bo Tang). J Hand Surg Eur 2014;39:107–15.

16. Tang JB, Amadio PC, Boyer MI, et al. Current practice of primary flexor tendon repair: A global view. Hand Clin 2013;29:179–89.

17. Lalonde DH. Conceptual origins, current practice, and views of wide awake hand surgery. J Hand Surg Eur 2017;42:886–95.

18. Wong JK, Peck F. Improving results of flexor tendon repair and rehabilitation. Plast Reconstr Surg 2014; 134:913e–25e.

19. Khor WS, Langer MF, Wong R, et al. Improving outcomes in tendon repair: A critical look at the evidence for flexor tendon repair and rehabilitation. Plast Reconstr Surg 2016;138:1045e–58e.

20. Tang JB. Rehabilitation after flexor tendon repair and others: a safe and efficient protocol. J Hand Surg Eur 2021;46:813–7.

21. Pan ZJ, Qin J, Zhou X, et al. Robust thumb flexor tendon repairs with a six-strand M-Tang method, pulley venting, and early active motion. J Hand Surg Eur 2017;42:909–14.

22. Giesen T, Sirotakova M, Copsey AJ, et al. Flexor pollicis longus primary repair: Further experience with the Tang technique and controlled active mobilization. J Hand Surg Eur 2009;34:758–61.

23. Chen J, Xian Zhang A, Jia Qian S, et al. Measurement of finger joint motion after flexor tendon repair: smartphone photography compared with traditional goniometry. J Hand Surg Eur 2021;46:825–9.

24. Pan ZJ, Xu YF, Pan L, et al. Zone 2 flexor tendon repairs using a tensioned strong core suture, sparse peripheral stitches and early active motion: results in 60 fingers. J Hand Surg Eur 2019;44:361–6.

25. Pan ZJ, Pan L, Xu YF, et al. Outcomes of 200 digital flexor tendon repairs using updated protocols and 30 repairs using an old protocol: experience over 7 years. J Hand Surg Eur 2020;45:56–63.

26. Prsic A, Bass JL, Moriya K, et al. Outcomes of release of the entire A4 pulley after flexor tendon repairs in Zone 2A followed by early active mobilization. J Hand Surg Eur 2016;41:400–5. Comment. 460.

27. Giesen T, Calcagni M, Elliot D. Primary flexor tendon repair with early active motion: experience in Europe. Hand Clin 2017;33:465–72.

28. Reissner L, Zechmann-Mueller N, Klein HJ, et al. Sonographic study of repair, gapping and tendon bowstringing after primary flexor digitorum profundus repair in zone 2. J Hand Surg Eur 2018;43: 480–6.

29. Lautenbach G, Guidi M, Tobler-Ammann B, et al. Six-strand flexor pollicis longus tendon repairs with and without circumferential sutures: a multicenter study. Hand (N Y) 2022. https://doi.org/10.1177/15589447211057295. 15589447211057295.

30. Frueh FS, Kunz VS, Gravestock IJ, et al. Primary flexor tendon repair in zones 1 and 2: early passive mobilization versus controlled active motion. J Hand Surg Am 2014;39:1344–50.

31. Lalonde DH. True active motion is superior to full fist place and hold after flexor tendon repair. J Hand Surg Eur 2019;44:866–7.

Surgical Considerations for Flexor Tendon Repair
Timing and Choice of Repair Technique and Rehabilitation

Sarah E. Sasor, MD[a],*, Kevin C. Chung, MD MS[b]

KEYWORDS

- Flexor tendon injury • Tendon laceration • Tendon repair • Tendon reconstruction
- Flexor tendon rehabilitation • Early active motion

KEY POINTS

- Surgical repair is essential for complete flexor tendon lacerations.
- Early repair (within 1 week) of flexor tendon lacerations is preferred.
- There are many acceptable flexor tendon repair techniques, most of which require a core suture with at least four strands and an epitendinous circumferential running suture.
- Tendon reconstruction is indicated in patients with segmental tendon loss or delayed presentation to care.
- Postoperative hand therapy is mandatory for optimal outcomes after flexor tendon surgery, and early active motion protocols are preferred.

INTRODUCTION

Flexor tendon injuries are common and occur mostly due to penetrating trauma. Surgical repair is required for complete tendon lacerations. The goal of surgical treatment is precise coaptation of the tendon ends with a strong repair that permits early active rehabilitation; this promotes tendon gliding, limits adhesion formation, and restores functional motion.

Outcomes after flexor tendon repair have improved significantly over the last 60 years with a better understanding of tendon biology and response to injury. Advancements in surgical techniques and rehabilitation protocols allow for good outcomes after early repair in all zones.

This article reviews the basics of tendon structure, function, healing, and anatomy. Repair techniques are discussed in detail for each flexor tendon zone. Postoperative rehabilitation greatly influences outcomes, and several protocols are described.

TENDON STRUCTURE AND FUNCTION

Microscopically, tendons are mostly composed of type 1 collagen and elastin embedded in a proteoglycan-water matrix. Macroscopically, healthy tendons are brilliant white and shiny with a fibroelastic texture. Tendons are surrounded by paratenon and epitenon, which together form a silky covering known as peritenon. Extra-synovial flexor tendons (zones 3–5) are surrounded by a collagenous, loose areolar-type tissue that aids in gliding and supports a complex microvascular network.[1]

Tendons have viscoelastic properties, including stress-relaxation and creep, and are highly deformable at low strain; this permits energy absorption during loading. High strain promotes

a Department of Plastic Surgery, Medical College of Wisconsin, Milwaukee, WI, USA; b Department of Surgery, Section of Plastic Surgery, University of Michigan, 1500 E. Medical Center Dr., 2130 Taubman Center, SPC 5340, Ann Arbor, MI 48109, USA
* Corresponding author. 1155 N Mayfair Rd, Suite T2600, Wauwatosa, WI 53226
E-mail address: ssasor@gmail.com

Hand Clin 39 (2023) 151–163
https://doi.org/10.1016/j.hcl.2022.08.016
0749-0712/23/© 2022 Elsevier Inc. All rights reserved.

tendon stiffness and facilitates the transmission of force from muscle to bone.[2]

Flexor tendon nutrition is supplied by an intrinsic and extrinsic vascular system. Intrinsic blood supply is provided by the vincula—folds of mesotenon that supply blood to the flexor digitorum superficialis (FDS) and flexor digitorum profundus (FDP) from the volar digital arteries.[3] There is some variation in vascular supply, but generally, flexor tendons have two vincula each that enter on the deep surface (**Fig. 1**). Extrinsic blood supply is provided by vessels that penetrate the tendon at muscle–tendon and bone–tendon interfaces, and smaller vessels that penetrate the peritenon from the surrounding areolar tissue. The extrinsic system is limited to tendon segments outside of the tendon sheath. Segments of tendon that are within the sheath are relatively avascular and rely on diffusion of nutrients from the synovial fluid.

Tenocyte synthetic function is both aerobic and anaerobic. Lower oxygen requirements permit tendons to maintain load for prolonged periods without sustaining ischemic damage; however, this also results in slow healing compared with muscle or bone.[4]

Tendon Healing

Phases of healing

Tendons heal via the typical phases of inflammation, proliferation, and remodeling:

- The inflammatory phase occurs during the first week and involves fibrin clot formation and the recruitment of inflammatory cells (neutrophils, macrophages, platelets, and erythrocytes). These cells facilitate neovascularization and stabilize the tendon ends within the zone of injury.[5]
- The proliferative phase occurs from 5 days to 4 weeks. Fibroblasts mediate the synthesis of proteoglycans, type 3 collagen, and other extracellular matrix components. Collagen formation is disorganized, and cell and water content increases.[6]

- Remodeling starts 1 month after repair and lasts for years. Cell and water content decreases and type 1 collagen is synthesized. Collagen reorganizes into longitudinal bundles along the tendon axis, which increases tendon strength.[7]

Cellular concepts

Historically, tendon healing has been classified into extrinsic and intrinsic processes depending on the presence or absence of a synovial sheath (zones 1 and 2). This concept oversimplifies the complex interplay of cells, gene expression, and growth factors but is useful in understanding the basic tenets of tendon healing.[8]

Extrinsic healing involves the invasion of fibroblasts and inflammatory cells from the surrounding synovium, paratenon, and tendon sheath into the site of injury. The extrinsic mechanism predominates early after tendon repair and is responsible for adhesions.

The intrinsic mechanism involves the tenocytes within the tendon itself. Tenocytes invade the defect and produce collagen, which reorganizes and aligns longitudinally to produce a healed tendon.[9,10] Movement of the tendon within the synovial sheath improves circulation and the delivery of nutrients. Intrinsic healing results in improved biomechanics and tendon gliding within the sheath.

The goal of tendon repair is to minimize extrinsic healing and maximize the intrinsic process. Early rehabilitation aims to reduce adhesion formation and enhance intrinsic remodeling.

Clinical healing

Practically speaking, the strength of a tendon immediately after repair is entirely reliant on the suture. Tendons are weakest during the early proliferative period (7 to 10 days) when initial deposition of disorganized type 3 collagen occurs. Tendon strength does not increase until the late proliferative period (after 21 days) when collagen remodeling begins. Remodeling takes months,

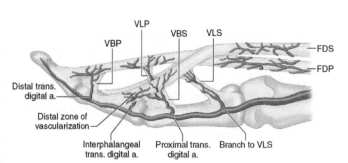

Fig. 1. Vascular supply to the flexor tendons. VBP, vincula brevus to profundus; VBS, vincula brevus to superficialis; VLP, vincular longus to profundus; VLS, vincular longus to superficialis. (*From* Chung K. Operative Techniques: Hand And Wrist Surgery (Fourth Edition). Elsevier; 2021; with permission.)

and unfortunately, never achieves complete regeneration; repaired tendons have thinner collagen fibrils with inferior strength and mechanical properties compared with uninjured tendons. Repaired tendons have 40% to 70% the strength of a normal tendon after complete healing.[11,12]

Surgical Anatomy

The FDS tendon inserts onto the base of the middle phalanx and functions to flex the proximal interphalangeal (PIP) joint. The FDP tendon inserts onto the base of the distal phalanx and acts as the primary flexor of the distal interphalangeal (DIP) joint, and as a secondary flexor of the PIP and metacarpophalangeal (MP) joints. The intrinsic muscles flex the MP joints and extend the PIP joints. The FDS tendon decussates at the level of the proximal phalanx to form Camper's chiasm, through which the FDP tendon passes (**Fig. 2**).

The thumb has a single proper extrinsic flexor tendon, the flexor pollicis longus (FPL) which originates on the radius and interosseous membrane and inserts onto the base of the distal phalanx.

Flexor tendon injuries are classified into five zones (**Fig. 3**):

Zone 1: Distal to the FDS insertion, contains only FDP.

Zone 2: Extends from the proximal aspect of A1 pulley to the FDS insertion. Contains both FDS and FDP tendons as they pass through the fibroosseus sheath.

Zone 3: Extends from distal aspect of carpal tunnel to the proximal aspect of the A1 pulley. The lumbricals originate from the radial aspect of the FDP tendons.

Zone 4: Proximal to distal aspect of carpal tunnel.

Zone 5: Extends from the musculotendinous junctions in the forearm to the proximal aspect of the carpal tunnel at the wrist crease.

Clinical Evaluation

History

Flexor tendon lacerations are often associated with other hand injuries, and a careful evaluation is mandatory. Take a detailed history including age, handedness, occupation, hobbies, general health, and previous hand injuries/surgeries. Clarify the mechanism of injury, hand position at the time of injury, and time elapsed since injury. Note current symptoms such as pain, altered sensation, and functional deficits. Patients with penetrating trauma should receive a tetanus booster if their previous dose was more than 5 years ago. If the wound is contaminated, consider administering antibiotics.

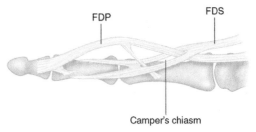

Fig. 2. Anatomy of FDS and FDP tendons in finger. (*From* Chung K. Operative Techniques: Hand And Wrist Surgery (Fourth Edition). Elsevier; 2021; with permission.)

Examination

Continuity of the FDS is evaluated by asking the patient to flex the finger, whereas the examiner holds the adjacent fingers in full extension (**Fig. 4**A). FDS to the small finger may be difficult to isolate and is anatomically absent in some patients.

The FDP tendon is evaluated by asking the patient to flex at the DIP joint with the PIP joint held in full extension (**Fig. 4**B).

The FPL tendon is examined by asking the patient to flex the interphalangeal joint of the thumb.

Imaging

Plain radiographs are required to evaluate for fractures and foreign bodies. A distal phalanx

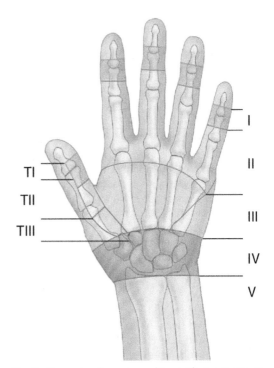

Fig. 3. Flexor tendon zones. (*From* Chung K. Operative Techniques: Hand And Wrist Surgery (Fourth Edition). Elsevier; 2021; with permission.)

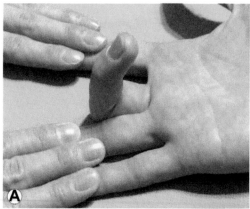

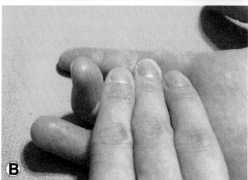

Fig. 4. Examination of the FDS (*A*) and FDP (*B*) tendons. (From Chung K. Operative Techniques: Hand And Wrist Surgery (Fourth Edition). Elsevier; 2021; with permission.)

avulsion fracture may indicate the location of the tendon stump if it remains attached to the tendon.

Preoperative Considerations

Indications

Flexor tendon repair is indicated in all patients with complete tendon lacerations who are medically stable for surgery. Repair of partial tendon lacerations is controversial but is generally recommended when more than 50% of the tendon is cut or if the cut end is triggering.[13–15]

Relative contraindications include severe contamination, unstable fractures, and segmental tendon loss.

Timing of repair

Flexor tendon repair in a perfused hand is not an emergency, and delay of up to 3 weeks in adults has been described.[16] However, with time, tendon ends become distorted, sheaths fibrose, adhesions form, and muscle–tendon units shorten, making repair and rehabilitation more difficult. Surgical repair within 1 week of injury is preferred.

Anesthesia

Surgery may be performed under local, regional, or general anesthesia depending on the complexity of the injury and patient/surgeon preference.

Flexor tendon repair under local anesthesia with epinephrine is safe and works well for cooperative patients. Wide-awake repair has several advantages over regional or general anesthesia. Patients can test the repair intraoperatively by flexing and extending the digit. Surgeons can check for bunching, gapping, and triggering and can revise the repair and vent pulleys as needed to ensure smooth active motion.

Brachial plexus blocks using supraclavicular, infraclavicular, or axillary approaches are all acceptable. General anesthesia is preferred for complex or multisystem injuries.

General Repair Principles

There are many nuances to tendon repair to optimize outcomes. General repair principles are as follows:

- Obtain adequate exposure using full thickness skin flaps.
- Preserve tendon blood supply.
- Preserve pulleys (when possible).
- Minimize direct tendon handling to avoid iatrogenic injury and grasp the corners of cut tendon ends with non-toothed forceps.
- Use a strong core suture construct with at least four strands.
- Create a smooth repair interface that prevents gap formation and minimizes bulkiness.

The strength of a tendon repair depends on the type and size of suture and the repair technique used. There are many acceptable techniques, most of which use a core suture and an epitendinous circumferential running suture.

Incisions

It is usually necessary to extend the laceration proximally and distally for adequate exposure during flexor tendon repair. Incisions should preserve flap vascularity and avoid crossing flexion creases at 90° to prevent postoperative contracture. The mid-axial approaches are preferred to preserve normal tissue directly over the tendon sheath. Bruner incisions are also acceptable (**Fig. 5**).

The distal tendon stump can usually be found within the wound after extending the incision distally. The proximal stump can often be retrieved by gently passing a mosquito through the flexor tendon sheath, flexing the wrist, and "milking" the tendon distally. If unsuccessful after one or two attempts, proximal incisions over the A1

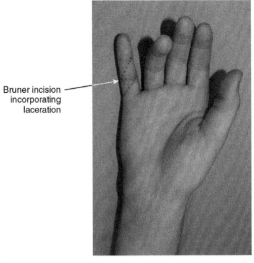

Fig. 5. Bruner incision. (*From* Chung K. Operative Techniques: Hand And Wrist Surgery (Fourth Edition). Elsevier; 2021; with permission.)

pulley, carpal tunnel, or flexor carpi radialis (FCR; for FPL tendon) are used.

Pulleys

The digital flexor tendon sheath is composed of five annular and three cruciate pulleys which hold the tendon close to the bone (**Fig. 6**). The A2 and

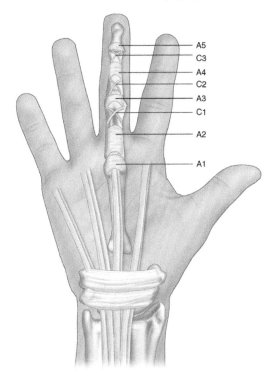

Fig. 6. Pulley system. (*From* Chung K. Operative Techniques: Hand And Wrist Surgery (Fourth Edition). Elsevier; 2021; with permission.)

A4 pulleys are critical in preventing bowstringing and decreasing the work of flexion.[17–19]

Venting pulleys adjacent to a tendon laceration is often necessary to obtain adequate purchase for core suture repair and to reduce constriction at the repair site. The pulleys are released just enough to allow for smooth gliding of the repair with full finger flexion and extension. Generally, if more than 50% of the A2 or A4 pulley is divided, pulley reconstruction is recommended; however, studies suggest that this may not be necessary if adjacent pulleys remain intact.[20]

Suture material

The ideal suture material for flexor tendon repair glides smoothly, has no memory or stretch, holds a knot, maintains tensile strength until intrinsic tendon healing occurs, and is biologically compatible. The biomechanical properties of suture materials have been extensively studied.[21,22] Each material has advantages and challenges, and ultimately, the choice of suture is based on surgeon preference. Common choices include synthetic monofilaments (Prolene or Ethilon), braided polyester (Ethibond), or newer materials such as braided, looped nylon (Supramid) or coated high molecular weight polyethylene (Fiberwire or Orthocord).

Synthetic monofilaments must be manually stretched to prevent postoperative elongation and gap formation. Monofilament sutures are difficult to handle and have poor knot security. Nonabsorbable polyester (Ethibond) is a braided alternative that has superior knot security and no tendency to stretch, but glides less and is difficult to evenly tension.

Bidirectional barbed suture (Quill) is a knotless option with similar tensile strength. Several ex vivo studies report adequate pull-out strength, but it has not been extensively studied clinically.[23]

Size 3 to 0 or 4 to 0 nonabsorbable suture on a tapered needle is used for flexor tendons in zones 1 to 5.

Core suture

The repair strength increases with the number of core strands, suture caliber, and purchase length; however, there is no high-level evidence that identifies the optimal number of core strands or repair technique. Increasing the number of core strands and suture caliber adds bulk to the repair which increases friction during tendon excursion; these goals must be balanced.

Biomechanical studies support the use of at least four core strands, with 7 to 10 mm of purchase, and dorsal suture placement (closer to the bone).[24–27] The knot should be buried within the core to reduce

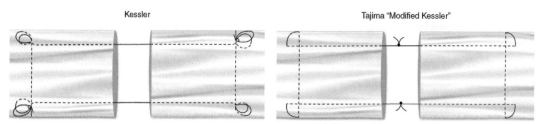

Fig. 7. Two-strand core techniques. (*From* Chung K. Operative Techniques: Hand And Wrist Surgery (Fourth Edition). Elsevier; 2021; with permission.)

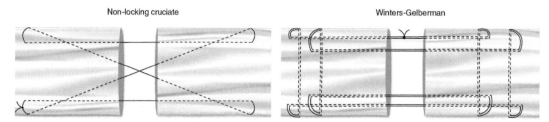

Fig. 8. Multistrand core techniques. (*From* Chung K. Operative Techniques: Hand And Wrist Surgery (Fourth Edition). Elsevier; 2021; with permission.)

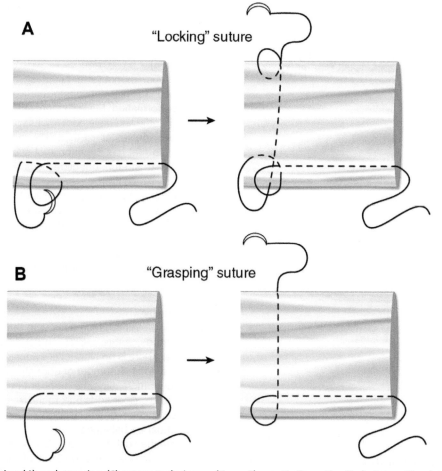

Fig. 9. Locking (*A*) and grasping (*B*) suture techniques. (*From* Chung K. Operative Techniques: Hand And Wrist Surgery (Fourth Edition). Elsevier; 2021; with permission.)

friction with motion. Many core suture repair techniques are described (**Figs. 7** and **8**).

Locking sutures are preferred over sliding (eg, Bunnell) or grasping (eg, cruciate, most modified Kessler) configurations as they facilitate increased transmission of axial tension (**Fig. 9**A,B).[28]

The authors prefer a six-strand Tang repair using a looped, braided suture or a Tajima-Strickland repair when looped suture is not available (**Fig. 10**A, B).

Epidendinous suture

Circumferential epitendinous repair reduces bulk at the repair site and increases the overall repair strength by up to 50%.[29] Strength can be increased by purchasing 2 to 3 mm from the tendon ends and increasing the depth of engagement (taking deeper bites). Size 5-0 or 6-0 synthetic monofilament suture on a tapered needle is used. Access to the dorsal flexor tendon can sometimes be optimized by completing the epitendinous repair before the core suture. Simple continuous or locking suture techniques are acceptable (**Fig. 11**). Epitendinous repair is recommended in zones 1 and 2 where tendon gliding is crucial and is optional for more proximal injuries.

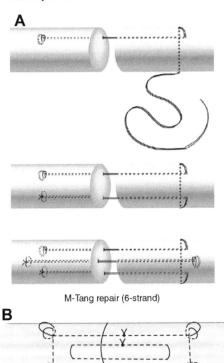

M-Tang repair (6-strand)

Fig. 10. M-Tang (*A*) and Tajima-Strickland (*B*) suture techniques. [A] *From* Tang JB, Zhou X, Pan ZJ, et al. Strong digital flexor tendon repair, extension-flexion test, and early active flexion: experience in 300 tendons. Hand Clin. 2017, 33:455–63; with permission.

Flexor Tendon Repair

Partial tendon injury

The treatment of partial tendon lacerations is controversial. Potential risks of untreated partial lacerations include symptomatic triggering, loss of excursion, or complete rupture. It is common practice to repair partial tendon lacerations of more than 50% of the cross-sectional area; however, studies show that this is not necessary and may be detrimental. Lacerations of up to 90% of the cross-sectional area can withstand the forces applied during rehabilitation.[30,31] In vivo suture repair of partial lacerations showed reduced tensile strength, higher rates of rupture, and less excursion compared with non-sutured, partially lacerated tendons.[32,33]

Partial flexor tendon lacerations may be debrided, and pulleys can be vented to prevent triggering. Near complete lacerations are treated with core and epitendinous sutures. The repair should be protected in a dorsal blocking splint and rehabilitated using active motion protocols akin to complete lacerations.

Complete injury

Zone 1 Zone 1 flexor tendon injuries involve only the FDP tendon and can result from a sharp laceration or an avulsion injury. Sharp lacerations can usually be repaired in a standard fashion if there is any distal stump present. Reinforcing sutures can be placed from the proximal tendon stump to the periosteum or A5 pulley as needed for very distal lacerations. Excursion is minimal near the tendon attachment on the distal phalanx, and the long-term functional goal is 30° to 40° of flexion at the DIP joint. When no distal stump is present, the tendon can be repaired using a pull-out button technique or bone anchor, as described below.

Avulsion injuries, also known as jersey fingers, occur when the finger is forcibly extended during active flexion. These injuries are uncommon and mostly occur in adolescents or young adults during sporting activities. The ring finger is most often affected. The avulsion can involve the tendon alone or the tendon and a fragment of distal

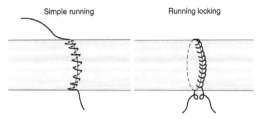

Simple running   Running locking

Fig. 11. Epitendinous suture. (*From* Chung K. Operative Techniques: Hand And Wrist Surgery (Fourth Edition). Elsevier; 2021; with permission.)

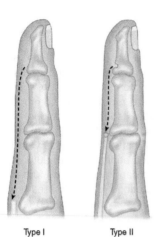
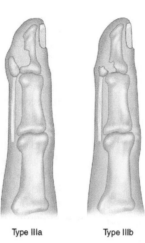

Type I   Type II   Type IIIa   Type IIIb

Fig. 12. Leddy–Packer classification for FDP avulsion injuries. (*From* Chung K. Operative Techniques: Hand And Wrist Surgery (Fourth Edition). Elsevier; 2021; with permission.)

phalanx. Leddy and Packer classified jersey fingers based on the presence of a fracture and the level of retraction of the proximal stump (**Fig. 12**).[34]

Type 1 injuries involve tendon avulsion from the distal phalanx without bony involvement. The vincula are disrupted, and the FDP retracts into the palm. Type 1 injuries require urgent repair due to the risk of tendon devascularization, pulley collapse, sheath fibrosis, and proximal muscle contracture. This type of injury has a worse prognosis because of the disruption to the vascular system.

Type 2 injuries involve a small bony avulsion and tendon retraction to the level of the PIP joint.

Type 3 injuries involve large (type 3A) or moderate (type 3B) avulsion fragments and tendon retraction to the level of the DIP joint.

Type 4 injuries are "double avulsion" injuries with an avulsion fracture and avulsion of the tendon from the fracture fragment, with subsequent retraction of the tendon into the palm.

Early repair is preferred for all avulsion injuries, but critical for Leddy–Packer types 1 and 4. This can be challenging as presentation is often delayed. Types 2 and 3 jersey fingers can be treated up to 3 months after the injury with good results.[35]

The fixation of the tendon to the distal phalanx is achieved using a pull-out button or bone anchor. For the pull-out button technique, a rongeur or curette is used to create a small corticotomy in the distal phalanx to expose cancellous bone for healing. A 3 to 0 nonabsorbable monofilament suture (Prolene) is passed through the distal tendon stump using a Bunnell-type suture (**Fig. 13**), and then passed through the distal phalanx using two parallel Keith needles. The Keith needles are driven antegrade and obliquely through the distal phalanx to exit through the sterile matrix or hyponychium (**Fig. 14**A, B). Care is taken to avoid drilling into the germinal matrix or lunula to prevent nail deformity (**Fig. 15**). The suture ends are tied over a button or felt pad on the nail plate under maximal tension (**Fig. 16**A–C). The tendon should be in direct contact with the bone with the suture tied. Multiple, square knots are advised.

Postoperatively, a splint is applied with the wrist in neutral, the MP joints flexed at 50° to 70°, and the IP joints in full extension. The button and suture material are removed 8 weeks postoperatively, and the gentle range of motion is initiated. Strengthening exercises are initiated at 12 weeks.

Some investigators report high complication rates with the pull-out suture technique including infection (22%), nail fold necrosis, nail plate deformity (35%), and DIP joint stiffness.[36] These can be minimized by creating a bone tunnel that exits distally on the nail plate and using a small button with a convex surface. Alternatively, bone anchors can be used to avoid an external button. Fluoroscopy should be used to confirm the anchor position. Care must be taken to avoid dorsal cortex violation to ensure proper seating of the anchor

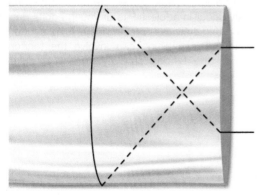

Fig. 13. Bunnell suture. (*From* Chung K. Operative Techniques: Hand And Wrist Surgery (Fourth Edition). Elsevier; 2021; with permission.)

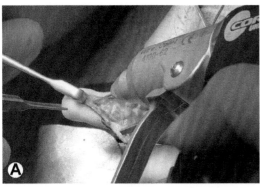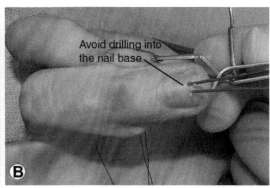

Fig. 14. Suture passed through the distal phalanx (*A, B*). (*From* Chung K. Operative Techniques: Hand And Wrist Surgery (Fourth Edition). Elsevier; 2021; with permission.)

and to protect the nail matrix. Bone anchors may have higher failure risks in osteoporotic bone and are contraindicated with large bony avulsion fragments.

Zone 1 flexor tendon repairs risk FDP overtightening resulting in quadriga–flexion lag in adjacent digits. The FDP tendons to the middle, ring, and small fingers share a common muscle belly, and the excursion of the combined tendons is equal to that of the shortest tendon. Advancement of the FDP tendon by more than 1 cm should be avoided.

Zone 2 Flexor tendon repairs in zone 2, also known as "no man's land," are unforgiving due to tenuous blood supply, a narrow fibro-osseous sheath, and the tendency for adhesion formation postoperatively. Repair is technically difficult due to the close relationship of FDS and FDP, Camper chiasm, and the pulley system. Bulky tendon repairs lead to friction, reduced tendon gliding, and postoperative stiffness. Outcomes following zone 2 repairs have improved significantly in recent decades with advances in suture material, improved repair techniques, and early active motion rehabilitation protocols.

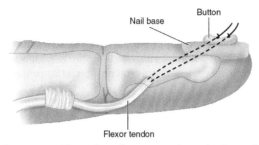

Fig. 15. Avoid passing the suture through the nail base. (*From* Chung K. Operative Techniques: Hand And Wrist Surgery (Fourth Edition). Elsevier; 2021; with permission.)

The repair of both the FDS and FDP tendons in zone 2 may cause overcrowding within the tendon sheath. When this occurs, three options exist:

1. Repair the FDP alone
2. Repair the FDP and a single slip of FDS
3. Repair both the FDP and FDS and vent the pulleys as needed to allow for smooth motion

Zones 3 to 5 Isolated tendon injures in Zones 3 to -5 are rare and concomitant injury to neurovascular structures should be excluded. Standard core suture repair techniques are used. Triggering in zone 3 may warrant release of the A1 pulley. In zone 4, carpal tunnel release should be performed to facilitate visualization and prevent compression of the median nerve. Zone 5 injuries often involve multiple tendons, the median and ulnar nerve, and the radial and ulnar arteries. Structures should be identified and systematically repaired.

Flexor pollicis longus Complete FPL lacerations in zones T1 and T2 are often associated with proximal stump retraction into the palm. When the tendon is not visible at the A1 pulley, a short, longitudinal incision is made overlying the FCR tendon in the distal forearm (**Fig. 17**). The FPL tendon is located just deep to the FCR. An 8-French pediatric feeding tube is passed through the tendon sheath from distal to proximal and sutured to the proximal tendon stump in the forearm wound. The feeding tube is pulled back out through the sheath and the tendon is delivered to the distal repair site (**Fig. 18**A, B).

Tendon Reconstruction

Tendon reconstruction is indicated in patients with segmental tendon loss or delayed presentation to care. Single-stage free tendon grafting is possible in patients with full passive range of motion, minimal scarring, an intact pulley system,

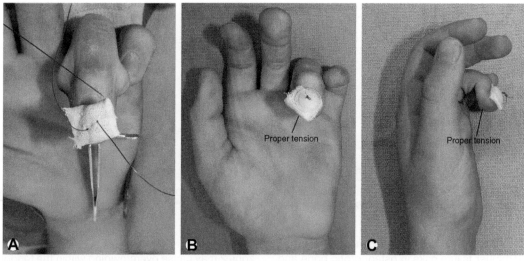

Fig. 16. Suture ends tied over a button on the nail plate under maximal tension (*A–C*). (*From* Chung K. Operative Techniques: Hand And Wrist Surgery (Fourth Edition). Elsevier; 2021; with permission.)

and no neurovascular involvement. Donor options include the palmaris longus, plantaris, and toe extensors.

A two-stage reconstruction is often necessary in injuries over 4 weeks old. Options include the

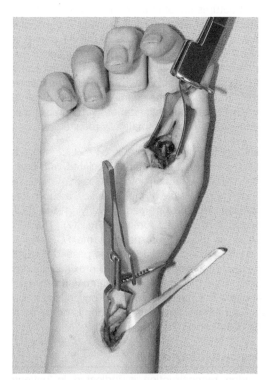

Fig. 17. FPL tendon is retrieved in the distal forearm through an incision over the radial FCR tendon. (*From* Chung K. Operative Techniques: Hand and Wrist Surgery (Fourth Edition). Elsevier; 2021; with permission.)

Hunter–Salisbury (free tendon graft) technique and the modified Paneva–Holovich technique (remnant FDS transposition).[37,38] Both techniques require debridement of the injured tendon and placement of a silicone spacer during the first stage. The silicone rod is sutured to the distal tendon stump and extended proximally into the palm or distal forearm. Pulleys are reconstructed as needed. A pseudosheath forms around the spacer over the course of 3 months which provides a smooth, gliding surface for the tendon graft in a second stage.

Tendon reconstruction is discussed in detail in, "Cathleen Cahill and colleagues "Women in Hand Surgery: Considerations and Support; A comprehensive review of the data, and important considerations including maternity, childcare, balance, and support for a career in hand surgery," of this issue.

REHABILITATION

Postoperative hand therapy is critical for optimal outcomes after flexor tendon repair. Patient understanding, motivation, and compliance are the key. Rehabilitation promotes intrinsic tendon healing, minimizes adhesions, and optimizes tendon gliding to restore functional motion while protecting the repair.

In the immediate postoperative period, a dorsal blocking splint is placed to prevent excessive tension on the repair. The splint should maintain the wrist in neutral, the MP joints flexed (50° to 70°), and the IP joints in slight flexion. Therapy is initiated 2 to 3 days postoperatively under the strict supervision of a certified hand therapist.

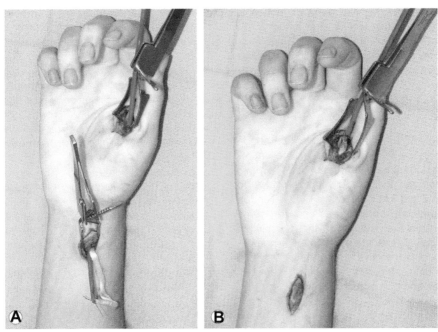

Fig. 18. Pediatric feeding tube is passed from distal to proximal through the tendon sheath and FPL stump is sutured to the end of the tube (*A*). Proximal FPL stump is delivered to the distal wound (*B*). (*From* Chung K. Operative Techniques: Hand And Wrist Surgery (Fourth Edition). Elsevier; 2021; with permission.)

Many therapy protocols exist. In general, they can be classified into three categories: (1) controlled passive motion, (2) place and hold, and (3) early active motion. There is some debate as to which strategy is the best.[39] The authors prefer early active motion protocols in compliant patients with strong repairs. Fractures, soft tissue injuries, and neurovascular repairs may also influence decision-making.

Early active protocols begin with active motion to a partial fist (50%), place and hold, and passive exercises within a dorsal blocking splint. These exercises enable differential gliding of the FDS and FDP tendons which decreases adhesion formation. Active motion is gradually increased over the next several weeks, and the wrist portion of the orthotic is removed at 4 weeks. Motion is increased in isolated joints. The dorsal blocking splint is discontinued, and strengthening is initiated 8 weeks postoperatively. Patients may return to full activity 3 to 4 months after surgery.

Patients who are unable to participate in early active hand therapy should begin the Duran protocol at their first postoperative visit. This passive motion plan was developed in the 1970s when two-strand repairs were common practice and is based on the theory that approximately 3 to 5 mm of tendon gliding is necessary to decrease

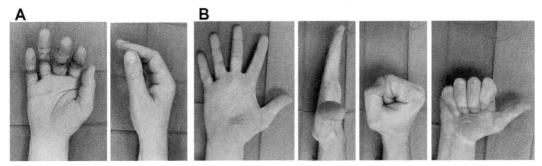

Fig. 19. (*A*) A 38-year-old man with laceration to the volar surface of the index, middle, ring, and small fingers. He underwent repair of the FDP to the index finger (zone 1), FDP and FDS to the middle finger (zone 2), FDP to the ring finger (zone 2), and FDP to the small finger (zone 2). He also had repairs of the several digital nerves and the ulnar digital artery to the small finger. (*B*) Seven months after surgery with early active motion rehabilitation.

adhesion formation. Passive range of motion is initiated in the first few weeks after surgery, followed by active motion starting at 4 weeks. Passive extension stretching and blocking exercises start at week 6, and strengthening begins 8 weeks postoperatively.

OUTCOMES

Approximately 80% of patients with flexor tendon repairs in zone 1 or 2 achieve good to excellent results (>75% normal total arc of motion) (**Fig. 19**A, B).[40] On average, the rate of rupture is 4% to 10% in zone 2 and 3 to 17% for the FPL.[41] Tendon adhesions and joint contractures occur in some patients and are likely related to the mechanism of injury, surgical technique, and patient compliance with postoperative rehabilitation. Close follow-up is critical for early recognition and intervention when complications occur.

CLINICS CARE POINTS

- Surgical repair is mandatory for complete flexor tendon lacerations.
- Repair flexor tendon lacerations within one week of injury.Surgical Care Points:
- Obtain adequate exposure using full thickness skin flaps.
- Preserve tendon blood supply.
- Preserve pulleys (when possible).
- Minimize direct tendon handling to avoid iatrogenic injury and adhesion formation.
- Use a strong core suture with at least four strands.
- Create a smooth repair interface that prevents gap formations and minimizes bulkiness.
- Post-operative hand therapy is essential for optimal outcomes.

DISCLOSURE

Kevin Chung receives funding from the National Institutes of Health, United States, book royalties from Wolters Kluwer and Elsevier, and a research grant from Sonex to study carpal tunnel outcomes.

REFERENCES

1. Guimberteau JC, Delage JP, Wong J. The role and mechanical behavior of the connective tissue in tendon sliding. Chir Main 2010;29(3):155–66.
2. Purslow PP, Wess TJ, Hukins DW. Collagen orientation and molecular spacing during creep and stress-relaxation in soft connective tissues. J Exp Biol 1998;201(Pt 1):135–42.
3. Ochiai N, Matsui T, Miyaji N, et al. Vascular anatomy of flexor tendons. I. Vincular system and blood supply of the profundus tendon in the digital sheath. J Hand Surg 1979;4(4):321–30.
4. Jozsa L, Balint JB, Reffy A, et al. Histochemical and ultrastructural study of adult human tendon. Acta Histochem 1979;65(2):250–7.
5. Lindsay WK, Birch JR. The fibroblast in flexor tendon healing. Plast Reconstr Surg 1964;34:223–32.
6. Garner WL, McDonald JA, Koo M, et al. Identification of the collagen-producing cells in healing flexor tendons. Plast Reconstr Surg 1989;83(5):875–9.
7. Liu SH, Yang RS, al-Shaikh R, et al. Collagen in tendon, ligament, and bone healing. A current review. Clin Orthop Relat Res 1995;(318):265–78.
8. Wu YF, Tang JB. Tendon healing, edema, and resistance to flexor tendon gliding: clinical implications. Hand Clin 2013;29(2):167–78.
9. Lundborg G, Rank F, Heinau B. Intrinsic tendon healing. A new experimental model. Scand J Plast Reconstr Surg 1985;19(2):113–7.
10. Lundborg G. Experimental flexor tendon healing without adhesion formation–a new concept of tendon nutrition and intrinsic healing mechanisms. A preliminary report. Hand 1976;8(3):235–8.
11. Maffulli N, Moller HD, Evans CH. Tendon healing: can it be optimised? Br J Sports Med 2002;36(5):315–6.
12. James R, Kesturu G, Balian G, et al. Tendon: biology, biomechanics, repair, growth factors, and evolving treatment options. J Hand Surg 2008;33(1):102–12.
13. Wray RC Jr, Holtman B, Weeks PM. Clinical treatment of partial tendon lacerations without suturing and with early motion. Plast Reconstr Surg 1977;59(2):231–4.
14. Wray RC Jr, Weeks PM. Treatment of partial tendon lacerations. Hand 1980;12(2):163–6.
15. Bishop AT, Cooney WP 3rd, Wood MB. Treatment of partial flexor tendon lacerations: the effect of tenorrhaphy and early protected mobilization. J Trauma 1986;26(4):301–12.
16. Schneider LH, Hunter JM, Norris TR, et al. Delayed flexor tendon repair in no man's land. J Hand Surg 1977;2(6):452–5.
17. Clark TA, Skeete K, Amadio PC. Flexor tendon pulley reconstruction. J Hand Surg 2010;35(10):1685–9.
18. Strickland JW. The scientific basis for advances in flexor tendon surgery. J Hand Ther 2005;18(2):94–110 [quiz: 111].
19. Doyle JR. Anatomy of the finger flexor tendon sheath and pulley system. J Hand Surg 1988;13(4):473–84.
20. Tang JB. Outcomes and evaluation of flexor tendon repair. Hand Clin 2013;29(2):251–9.

21. Trail IA, Powell ES, Noble J. An evaluation of suture materials used in tendon surgery. J Hand Surg Br 1989;14(4):422–7.

22. Lawrence TM, Davis TR. A biomechanical analysis of suture materials and their influence on a four-strand flexor tendon repair. J Hand Surg 2005;30(4):836–41.

23. Shah A, Rowlands M, Au A. Barbed sutures and tendon repair-a review. Hand (N Y). 2015;10(1):6–15.

24. Cao Y, Zhu B, Xie RG, et al. Influence of core suture purchase length on strength of four-strand tendon repairs. J Hand Surg 2006;31(1):107–12.

25. Bernstein MA, Taras JS. Flexor tendon suture: a description of two core suture techniques and the Silfverskiold epitendinous suture. Tech Hand Up Extrem Surg 2003;7(3):119–29.

26. Tang JB, Zhang Y, Cao Y, et al. Core suture purchase affects strength of tendon repairs. J Hand Surg 2005;30(6):1262–6.

27. Soejima O, Diao E, Lotz JC, et al. Comparative mechanical analysis of dorsal versus palmar placement of core suture for flexor tendon repairs. J Hand Surg 1995;20(5):801–7.

28. Tanaka T, Amadio PC, Zhao C, et al. Gliding characteristics and gap formation for locking and grasping tendon repairs: a biomechanical study in a human cadaver model. J Hand Surg 2004;29(1):6–14.

29. Diao E, Hariharan JS, Soejima O, et al. Effect of peripheral suture depth on strength of tendon repairs. J Hand Surg 1996;21(2):234–9.

30. Lineberry KD, Shue S, Chepla KJ. The management of partial zone II intrasynovial flexor tendon lacerations: a literature review of biomechanics, clinical outcomes, and complications. Plast Reconstr Surg 2018;141(5):1165–70.

31. Hariharan JS, Diao E, Soejima O, et al. Partial lacerations of human digital flexor tendons: a biomechanical analysis. J Hand Surg 1997;22(6):1011–5.

32. Ollinger H, Wray RC Jr, Weeks PM. Effects of suture on tensile strength gain of partially and completely severed tendons. Surg Forum 1975;26:63–4.

33. Reynolds B, Wray RC Jr, Weeks PM. Should an incompletely severed tendon be sutured? Plast Reconstr Surg 1976;57(1):36–8.

34. Leddy JP, Packer JW. Avulsion of the profundus tendon insertion in athletes. J Hand Surg 1977;2(1):66–9.

35. Kang N, Pratt A, Burr N. Miniplate fixation for avulsion injuries of the flexor digitorum profundus insertion. J Hand Surg Br 2003;28(4):363–8.

36. Kang N, Marsh D, Dewar D. The morbidity of the button-over-nail technique for zone 1 flexor tendon repairs. Should we still be using this technique? J Hand Surg Eur 2008;33(5):566–70.

37. Hunter JM, Salisbury RE. Flexor-tendon reconstruction in severely damaged hands. A two-stage procedure using a silicone-dacron reinforced gliding prosthesis prior to tendon grafting. J Bone Joint Surg Am 1971;53(5):829–58.

38. Paneva-Holevich E. Two-stage tenoplasty in injury of the flexor tendons of the hand. J Bone Joint Surg Am 1969;51(1):21–32.

39. Thien TB, Becker JH, Theis JC. Rehabilitation after surgery for flexor tendon injuries in the hand. Cochrane Database Syst Rev 2004;4:CD003979.

40. Tang JB. Clinical outcomes associated with flexor tendon repair. Hand Clin 2005;21(2):199–210.

41. Dy CJ, Hernandez-Soria A, Ma Y, et al. Complications after flexor tendon repair: a systematic review and meta-analysis. J Hand Surg 2012;37(3):543–551 e541.

Tips to Successful Flexor Tendon Repair and Reconstruction with WALANT

Donald H. Lalonde, FRCSC[a],*, Sarvnaz Sepehripour, MD[b]

KEYWORDS

- WALANT flexor tendon surgery • WALANT tendon grafting • WALANT one stage tendon grafting
- WALANT tenolysis • Pulley venting A2 and A4 • Intraoperative patient education

KEY POINTS

- To decrease adhesions and the need for tenolysis in flexor tendon repair, WALANT has taught us that we need to vent enough of any pulley to permit free gliding of the repair from full fist active flexion to full active extension during surgery by the awake patient.
- In WALANT flexor tendon repair, you can see gaps that appear with active flexion if the sutures are not tight enough. Gaps would lead to rupture if not seen and repaired during surgery. Gapping and rupture are less likely with a bulky repair that easily fits between unvented pulleys.
- In flexor tendon tenolysis, the surgeon and the patient take turns working on the adhesions with surgical dissection and with patient active flexion that pulls the tendon out of scar.
- In flexor tendon reconstruction, WALANT shows that we can easily and successfully reuse the A2 pulley that is buried in scar to permit 1-stage flexor reconstruction with a flexor digitorum superficialis flexor tendon graft.
- Intraoperative patient education of the unsedated patients has been found to be very effective in decreasing postoperative rupture and adhesions because of increased patient compliance.

 Video content accompanies this article at http://www.hand.theclinics.com.

CLINICS CARE POINTS FOR GOOD RESULTS IN FLEXOR TENDON REPAIR

- Surgeons should perform their own ultrasound before surgery to locate tendon ends accurately and shorten incisions.
- Short finger incisions with a separate palm incision, if necessary, decrease postoperative scarring, adhesions, and the likelihood of tenolysis.
- Take 1 cm bites of tendon on both sides for a good solid suture and repair.
- Use a minimum of 4 strands in the repair. The 6-strand M-Tang repair is preferable.
- A bulky repair that fits through vented pulleys decreases the risk of gapping and rupture.

- WALANT full fist flexion and extension testing reveals gaps so the surgeon can repair them to prevent rupture.
- WALANT full fist flexion and extension testing ensures adequate pulley venting to avoid tenolysis.
- Up to 1.5 to 2 cm of total pulley venting, including A2 or A4, if necessary, to allow full glide of the repair from unvented pulley proximally in full fist flexion to unvented pulley distally in full fist extension by the awake unsedated patient.
- Intraoperative education of the patient by the surgeon during WALANT repair decreases the risk of postoperative rupture, infection, and tenolysis.

[a] Dalhousie University, Suite C204, 600 Main Street, Saint John, NB E2K 1J5, Canada; [b] Birmingham Women's and Children's National Health Service Foundation Trust, Steelhouse Lane, Birmingham, England B4 6NH, UK
* Corresponding author.
E-mail address: dlalonde@drlalonde.ca

Hand Clin 39 (2023) 165–170
https://doi.org/10.1016/j.hcl.2022.08.017

- Elevation and immobilization for 3 to 5 days after surgery to let the swelling settle and give time for patients to get off all pain medication so they can do pain-guided therapy.
- After 3 to 5 days, when collagen formation starts, start up to half a fist of early protected, pain-guided, true active movement.
- If repair gets stuck in scar in the weeks after surgery, the surgeon performs ultrasound to verify that the repair is not ruptured and asks the hand therapist to start relative motion extension splinting or CMMS (casting motion to mobilize stiffness).

CLINICS CARE POINTS FOR LOCAL ANESTHESIA INJECTION PRINCIPLES

- Inject the patient lying down on a stretcher to decrease the risk of fainting.
- The goal of tumescent local anesthesia is to have the entire area of dissection tumesced 2 cm beyond any area of dissection.
- Tumescence means that all subcutaneous tissue to be dissected is swollen with visible and palpable local anesthesia.
- If you limit your volume to 50 mL of 1% lidocaine with epinephrine you do not need to monitor the patient[1] and you can perform the surgery outside the main operating room for patient and surgeon convenience.
- Always wait for 30 minutes or more between injection and surgery to give epinephrine hemostasis and lidocaine numbness time to work well.
- Inject patients outside the operating room before they come in to give local anesthesia time to work.
- Use well-documented minimal pain injection techniques so patients thing you are magical.[2]

TO DECREASE THE PAIN OF LOCAL ANESTHESIA INJECTION FOR WALANT FLEXOR TENDON REPAIR[3]

- Buffer acidic 1% lidocaine with 1:100,000 epinephrine with 8.4% bicarbonate (10 mL:1 mL) to decrease the acidity sting.[4]
- Start with a half-inch 30-gauge half-inch needle on a 3-mL syringe to decrease the first needle poke sting.
- Before needle insertion, have the thumb ready on the plunger and the syringe stabilized with both hands to decrease unnecessary pain from needle movement in the skin until it gets numb.[5]

- Warn the patient to try not to move when they feel the needle go in to avoid having to poke them twice because they moved.
- Create sensory noise by pressing on the skin very firmly just proximal to the needle insertion site at the time of insertion.
- Ask the patient to take a deep breath and insert the needle at mid-inspiration.
- Inject the first 2 to 3 mL of local anesthesia just under the skin without moving the needle at all.
- Always reinsert or advance needles in clearly numb skin so all the patient feels is the first poke of the first needle.
- When needle advancement is required, always inject antegradely while slowly advancing from proximal to distal.
- When needle reinsertion is required, always reinsert 1 cm inside the tumesced border of clearly numbed skin to eliminate needle reinsertion pain. Alternate between radial and ulnar reinsertion points.
- Always inject from proximal to distal to take advantage of distal nerves already being numbed by proximally injected local anesthesia.
- Give the lidocaine with epinephrine local anesthesia 30 minutes or more to work to ensure numbness and optimal hemostasis.

ULTRASOUND EXAMINATIONS BY THE SURGEON BEFORE AND AFTER SURGERY

Doing your own ultrasound lets you know exactly where the tendon ends are so you can make shorter incisions (Video 1). The shorter the incisions, the less the postoperative scarring with adhesions that might lead to unnecessary tenolysis.

When we see patients in the clinic for their rehabilitation, we let them watch their own tendons move as they hold the ultrasound probe over their finger for instant feedback.

If active dip movement stops in the weeks after surgery, you can easily see profundus with ultrasound to know instantly if it has ruptured or just got stuck in scar formation. Rupture is clearly an indication to return to surgery. If the tendons are stuck in scar, we like to start relative motion extension splinting.[6]

ADDITIONAL TIPS FOR PLANNING AND LOCAL INJECTION FOR FLEXOR TENDON REPAIR IN THE FINGER OR HAND

Plan the shortest incisions possible to decrease postoperative scarring, adhesions, and the need for tenolysis. Your preoperative ultrasound examination will tell you exactly where the tendon ends are located. Plan a separate small incision in the palm to push the tendon distally with 2 Adson forceps like a rope if this is required.

For a 3-finger flexor repair you will need 30 mL of buffered 1% lidocaine with 1:100,000 epinephrine.

For one finger you will need 10 to 15 mL of local.

Start by injecting 10 mL in the part of the palm or wrist where you are most likely to need to dissect the most proximally. Add 2 mL in the middle of the phalanx in the subcutaneous fat of each proximal and middle phalanx. Do not inject in the flexor tendon sheath. For Zone 1, you can add no more than 0.5 mL in the distal phalanx proximal pulp, but this is usually unnecessary because of the 2 mL of local you have injected in the middle phalanx.

SPECIFICS OF SUTURING, PULLEY VENTING, AND TESTING OF THE REPAIR

We prefer a 4-0 braided nylon looped suture 6-strand M-Tang repair, which is 10-20% bulky.[7] The bites need to be generous at 1 cm from the tendon cut. The knots should be outside the repair, so they do not impair tendon healing at the repair site.[8] WALANT has shown us that knots outside of a properly vented flexor tendon sheath do not restrict repair gliding.

Do not be afraid to have the patient test the repair with full fist active flexion and extension several times during the surgery. If you do these in the main operating room, take down the "sterile" drape so the patient can see his finger during this part of the repair testing. He has no idea where his finger is in space because it is numb. He can only follow your instructions to move his fingers if he can see at least his fingertip. You can cover the wound if required so he does not see raw tissue.

You need to test the repair to make sure it glides freely from unvented proximal pulley to unvented distal pulley, even if that means venting the A2 or A4 pulley if necessary.[9] The old "never vent A2 or A4" rule has been replaced with the new guideline to judiciously vent up to a total of 1.5 to 2 cm of the pulleys[10] (**Fig. 1** and Video 2).

You also need to test the repair to make sure there is no gapping with the forces of active flexion and extension. Gapping occurs 7% of the time and will lead to rupture if not corrected at the time of surgery.[11]

HOW TO REPAIR A GAP THAT OCCURS WHEN THE REPAIR IS TESTED DURING WALANT SURGERY

- Do not remove the first gapping suture that has been demonstrated to be too loose with active flexion. You can tighten and reuse the

first suture where it is, so you do not add further tendon trauma by reinserting it.
- Put in a second tighter suture but leave the 2 suture ends long when you tie the knot.
- Now you can tighten the first loose suture by pulling on one of its loops or its knot until it is as tight as it should be.
- Take the loose loop or knot of the first tightened suture and tie it to the long ends of the second suture.

EPITENON SUTURES

Watching repaired flexor tendons move at surgery has moved us away from thinking that epitenon sutures are necessary to add strength. The repair is plenty strong if made bulky with a 6-strand M-Tang repair.

The epitenon is a major source of tendon healing cells. We therefore do not want to strangle epitenon blood supply any more than we want to strangle skin blood supply when we suture facial lacerations. Our goal is to have both sides of the epitenon kissing gently along the entire repair border without being strangled. This will facilitate cell migration and healing in the gap.

We therefore wait until the core sutures are placed and tested several times with active flexion and extension. We examine the appearance of the epitenon with this movement. We then place sutures only where they are needed to accomplish the goal of gently touching cells at the border of the repair.

PARTIAL TENDON LACERATIONS

Partial tendon lacerations of up to 90% can be managed case by case as seen by examining active movement at the time of surgical exploration without necessarily having to formally repair the lacerated portions.[12]

INTRAOPERATIVE EDUCATION

Flexor tendon surgery changes patients' lives radically for the month after surgery. Patients are frequently unprepared for these changes and do not alter their activities enough to decrease the risks of postoperative complications such as rupture.

Surgeons who regularly do WALANT tendon surgery have found that one-on-one intraoperative education of the patient by the surgeon is very helpful in modifying postoperative activity (Video 3).

We explain to each and every patient how important elevation, immobilization, and pain-guided healing are to eliminate swelling, the use of pain medication, and the work of flexion in the first 3 to 5 days after surgery. The patients know from the intraoperative surgeon education that "I

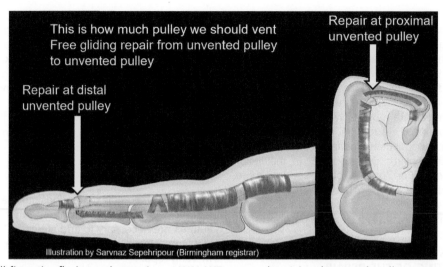

This is how much pulley we should vent
Free gliding repair from unvented pulley
to unvented pulley

Repair at distal
unvented pulley

Repair at proximal
unvented pulley

Illustration by Sarvnaz Sepehripour (Birmingham registrar)

Fig. 1. Full fist active flexion and extension at WALANT surgery determines how much pulley we need to vent. The slightly bulky repair needs to glide freely from distal unvented pulley to proximal unvented pulley with active patient flexion and extension during the surgery. (*Courtesy of* Sarvnaz Sepehripour, MD, Birmingham, England.)

can move it, but I can't use it" with early protected movement. They also understand that they will not need to do more than half a fist of active movement to decrease the risk of rupture. They know that they will need to keep it moving so it does not get stuck in scar.

Sedated patients may not remember anything. The best sedation for education is no sedation.

POSTOPERATIVE THERAPY CHANGES BROUGHT ABOUT BY WALANT

Intraoperative simulation of "full fist place and hold" (Duran) postoperative therapy (passive flexion followed by asking the patient to maintain flexion) does not always result in the flexor tendon moving with passive finger flexion. Instead of passively moving, the repaired tendon can simply buckle. As a result, when we ask the unsedated patient to maintain the flexion during the surgery, the repair can jerk into full flexion; this is demonstrated in the videos accessible in the open access reference on this subject.[13] Half a fist of true active protected pain-guided movement does not jerk and is a more natural movement. It is therefore more attractive as a postoperative therapy regimen than full fist passive flexion followed by active flexion (place and hold).[14]

WALANT SPAGHETTI WRIST REPAIRS

Prepare 100 mL of 0.5% lidocaine with 1:200,000 epinephrine by adding 50 mL of saline to 50 mL of buffered lidocaine with epinephrine. After you raise the skin flaps, first identify the proximal nerve stumps. With fine forceps, pick up the epineurium

of large median and ulnar nerves without painfully touching the proximal live fascicles. Inject 3 to 5 mL of local anesthesia just inside the epineurium so the loose areolar tissue around the fascicles bulges as a hot dog on a stick for 1 to 2 cm proximal to the lacerated nerve stump. Give time for the proximal nerve ends get numb while you do all the tendon work. The nerves are numb by the time you are ready to coapt them.

We use the above nerve numbing strategy because it has been shown that large nerves such as the median nerve at the wrist level can take 100 minutes for the local anesthesia to penetrate the center of the nerve if only the outside of the nerve is bathed with 1% lidocaine.[15]

Sometimes it is hard to match proximal and distal tendon ends; this is especially true with ragged cuts such as table saw injuries. There are 2 good WALANT strategies to help identify the correct proximal tendon ends. The first is to pull on a proximal tendon and ask the patient which "finger" you are pulling on. The unsedated patient feels the muscle belly proprioceptive nerves fire in the ring "finger" flexors when you pull on the ring finger proximal tendon. The second strategy is to ask the patient to flex his ring finger. The ring finger proximal tendon stump moves more than the other tendon stumps when the patient does this.

WALANT FLEXOR TENDON TENOLYSIS

With tenolysis, local anesthesia does not cross scar lines easily because scarring creates a barrier to diffusion of local anesthesia. A good strategy to inject local anesthesia for these cases is to start generous injections proximal to any scars where the local anesthesia can diffuse easily (Video 4). Then you can inject on both sides of existing scars, alternating from radial to ulnar, always reinserting needles into numb areas.[16] All areas to be dissected need to be bathed with tumescent local anesthesia.

We prefer to release the tendon from the sheath via sheathotomy. We use a Freer elevator on the palmar surface and sides of the tendon. Sharp Steven tenotomy scissor dissection is more helpful on the bone side of the flexors to free adhesions around the vinculae. After the tendons seem to be free to the surgeon's eye, we ask the patient to help us by flexing forcefully. Take down the drapes. He needs to see his finger to do this because it is numb, and he does not know where it is in space. The patient will frequently rupture the last little bit of adhesions. Sometimes, they feel their adhesions rupture in the wrist, even when we think the adhesions were all in the finger.

Seeing a very slim tendon repair move at the end of tenolysis surgery has also changed our postoperative therapy regimen. We can see that the tendon repair has been robbed of all its external collagen strength, as well as most of its external blood supply. The tenolysed tendon is very weak and prone to rupture. We therefore treat it just like a freshly repaired flexor tendon with 3 to 5 days of immobilization and elevation followed by up to half a fist of protected pain-guided true active movement, so it does not get stuck while it gains healing strength.

WALANT FLEXOR GRAFTING

Prepare 200 mL of 0.25% lidocaine with 1:400,000 epinephrine by adding 150 mL of saline to 50 mL of 1% lidocaine with 1:100,000 epinephrine. Always inject local proximal to distal, alternating between radial and ulnar when the needle is reinserted. Inject proximal enough that flexor digitorum superficialis (FDS) can be harvested as a tendon graft to bridge the profundus gap. We prefer to use FDS as a donor graft. The FDP proximal stump can be observed to actively move with flexion by the awake unsedated patient. If there is 2 cm of movement of the proximal FDP stump after it is liberated from scar, it will be a useful motor.

WALANT has shown us that 1-stage flexor tendon repair by using the original A2 pulley dug out of scar can work well (see Video 5) and save the patient from the extra operation and complications of 2-stage flexor tendon repairs with Hunter implants (rods). The same injection principles can be followed in both stages of a 2-stage WALANT flexor tendon reconstruction, but the we prefer 1-stage tendon grafting.

SUMMARY

This article reviews important recent changes WALANT has facilitated in flexor tendon reconstruction. These changes include the following: (1) proper pulley venting of even A2 or A4; (2) intraoperative full fist active flexion and extension testing by the patient to avoid rupture and tenolysis; (3) intraoperative patient education by the surgeon to decrease postoperative complications; (4) 1-stage flexor tendon grafting with FDS donor tendons through the original A2 pulley tunneled under the scar; (5) patient active assisted tenolysis; (6) proximal tendon identification strategies in spaghetti wrist; (7) true active movement instead of full fist place and hold for postoperative therapy; (8) the elimination of the need for sedation and the tourniquet with new minimal pain local anesthesia injection techniques; and (9) ultrasound examination by the surgeon preoperatively for shorter scars and postoperatively to distinguish rupture from adhesions stopping profundus glide.

DISCLOSURE

Dr Lalonde receives consulting fees from ASSI instruments.

Dr Lalonde is the editor of 2 books. All of the royalties from both the first and second editions of Wide Awake Hand Surgery go to the lean and green effort, which is dedicated to promoting less unnecessary cost and trash production in hand surgery.

SUPPLEMENTARY DATA

Supplementary data related to this article can be found online at https://doi.org/10.1016/j.hcl.2022.08.017.

REFERENCES

1. Farkash U, Herman A, Kalimian T, et al. Keeping the finger on the pulse: cardiac arrhythmias in hand surgery using local anesthesia with adrenaline. Plast Reconstr Surg 2020;146(1):54e–60e.
2. Joukhadar N, Lalonde D. How to minimize the pain of local anesthetic injection for wide awake surgery. Plast Reconstr Surg Glob Open 2021;9(8):e3730.
3. Lalonde DH. Chapter 5 how to inject local anesthesia so that it does not hurt. In: Lalonde DH, editor. Wide awake hand surgery and therapy tips. 2nd edition. New York: Thieme publishers; 2021. p. 43–55.
4. Frank SG, Lalonde DH. How acidic is the lidocaine we are injecting, and how much bicarbonate should we add? Can J Plast Surg 2012;20(2):71–3.

5. Strazar AR, Leynes PG, Lalonde DH. Minimizing the pain of local anesthesia injection. Plast Reconstr Surg 2013;132(3):675–84.

6. Tang JB, Xing SG, Wong J, et al. Chapter 19 flexor tendon repair of the finger. In: Lalonde DH, editor. Wide awake hand surgery and therapy tips. 2nd edition. New York: Thieme Publishers; 2021. p. 155–76.

7. Tang JB. New developments are improving flexor tendon repair. Plast Reconstr Surg 2018;141(6):1427–37.

8. Tang JB, Lalonde D, Harhaus L, et al. Flexor tendon repair: recent changes and current methods. J Hand Surg Eur 2022;47(1):31–9.

9. Moriya K, Yoshizu T, Tsubokawa N, et al. Clinical results of releasing the entire A2 pulley after flexor tendon repair in zone 2C. J Hand Surg Eur 2016;41(8):822–8.

10. Tang JB, Zhou X, Pan ZJ, et al. Strong digital flexor tendon repair, extension-flexion test, and early active flexion: experience in 300 tendons. Hand Clin 2017;33(3):455–63.

11. Higgins A, Lalonde DH, Bell M, et al. Avoiding flexor tendon repair rupture with intraoperative total active movement examination. Plast Reconstr Surg 2010;126(3):941–5.

12. Lineberry KD, Shue S, Chepla KJ. The management of partial zone II intrasynovial flexor tendon lacerations: a literature review of biomechanics, clinical outcomes, and complications. Plast Reconstr Surg 2018;141(5):1165–70.

13. Meals C, Lalonde D, Candelier G. Repaired flexor tendon excursion with half a fist of true active movement versus full fist place and hold in the awake patient. Plast Reconstr Surg Glob Open 2019;7(4):e2074.

14. Lalonde D. True active motion is superior to full fist place and hold after flexor tendon repair. J Hand Surg Eur 2019;44(8):866–7.

15. Lovely LM, Chishti YZ, Woodland JL, et al. How much volume of local anesthesia and how long should you wait after injection for an effective wrist median nerve block? Hand (N Y) 2018;13(3):281–4.

16. Wong J, Saurbier M, Amadio P, et al. Chapter 23 tenolysis. In: Lalonde DH, editor. Wide awake hand surgery and therapy tips. 2nd edition. New York: Thieme Publishers; 2021. p. 203–8.

Flexor Tendon Adhesion Formation: Current Concepts

Tomoyuki Kuroiwa, MD, PhD, Peter C. Amadio, MD*

KEYWORDS

- Tendon adhesion • Tendon repair • Tendon injury • Lubricin • Biomaterials • TGF-Beta • Hydrogel
- PXL01

KEY POINTS

- Methods of preventing tendon adhesions have been studied for more than 50 years, and various physical and chemical/biological methods have been proposed.
- Except for early motion, most of these methods have shortcomings or have failed to demonstrate efficacy in clinical studies and are still not used at the routine clinical level.
- Animal studies with Lubricin and PXL01 have shown a reduction in adhesion formation without adverse effects on tendon repair, and further clinical studies are planned.
- In addition, biocompatible biomaterials containing chemical/molecular biological components have been developed in recent years. This gives us hope that innovative methods to reduce adhesions will emerge that can be used in clinical practice.

INTRODUCTION/HISTORY/DEFINITIONS/BACKGROUND

Tendon adhesions are the most common complication in finger flexor tendon repair.[1] Adhesions, in which a tendon attaches to the surrounding tissue, reduce the normal gliding ability of the tendon and causes a partial loss of range of motion (ROM) of the finger. Adhesion formation after injury to intrasynovial tendons, such as the finger flexors, is a complex problem because it is part of the tendon healing process and occurs almost inevitably as a physiologic response to tendon injury.[2] This is further complicated by the fact that intrasynovial tendons are hypocellular (**Fig. 1**) and depend on a mixture of synovial and segmental vascular nutrition for sustenance. The cells that ultimately join the lacerated tendon ends to heal the tendon injury originate from the epitenon, which is topologically contiguous with the tendon sheath. As this cell layer is activated in response to injury, it is impossible currently to isolate the healing of the tendon from the healing of tissues that envelop the tendon, even in a sharply lacerated wound.[3] The result is often a healed tendon that is also healed to its synovial sheath, resulting in limited

motion and functional loss. This is especially true if the tendon blood supply has been injured as well. An ischemic tendon will inevitably require an ingrowth of adhesions to heal.[4]

During the past decades, numerous methods have been developed to reduce and minimize adhesion formation. One effective method has been the development of suture repair techniques that are less traumatic, less bulky, and thus less likely to cause inflammation or interfere with tendon gliding postoperatively. Such repairs are less prone to adhesion formation. Judicious pulley excision can also improve tendon gliding postoperatively and thus reduce the risk of motion-limiting adhesions. Even more important has been the development of early mobilization and low force rehabilitation methods.[5] Other attempts have been less successful. Lubricants such as hyaluronic acid (HA) have been used to prevent adhesions. In addition, physical barriers have been used to prevent adhesions, as have biologically active compounds to reduce scar tissue formation.[6] Again, the trick (yet to be identified in practice) is how to block healing *around* the tendon, without also blocking healing *within* the tendon. Most recently, research has been conducted into

Department of Orthopedic Surgery, Mayo Clinic, 200 First St. SW, Rochester, MN, USA
* Corresponding author.
E-mail address: pamadio@mayo.edu

0749-0712/23/© 2022 Elsevier Inc. All rights reserved.

hand.theclinics.com

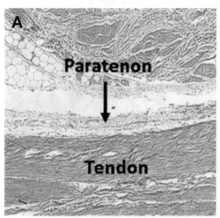 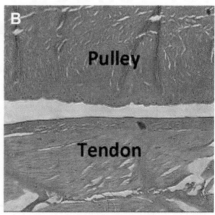

Extrasynovial   Intrasynovial

Fig. 1. Histology of extrasynovial tendon (*A*) and intrasynovial tendon (*B*). The intrasynovial tendon does not have a paratenon along it and is hypocellular. (*From* Amadio PC. Gliding resistance and modifications of gliding surface of tendon: clinical perspectives. Hand Clinics. 2013;29(2):159–166; with permission.)

the development of advanced technologies that combine both functions, such as biomaterials for tendon repair site protection that can release externally facing adhesion-reducing chemicals while simultaneously delivering (or protecting) cells and growth factors internally to promote healing of the tendon ends. Similar technology is now in use clinically to promote primary repair of knee anterior cruciate ligaments.[7] This article will review the current state of knowledge regarding tendon adhesion formation, prevention, and future research directions.

FROM INJURY TO TENDON ADHESION FORMATION

When a tendon is injured, inflammation and angiogenesis occur in and around the injured tendon. This process is essentially identical in all soft tissues. During this process, transforming growth factor-beta (TGF-β), which is present in small amounts in the original uninjured tendon and surrounding tendon sheath, is increased in its expression and production in tenocytes, infiltrating fibroblasts, and inflammatory cells.[8,9] In particular, of the 3 isoforms of TGF-β, TGF-β1 has been most associated with adhesion formation.[10] Maeda and colleagues also reported that TGF-β1 release occurs after tendon injury due to the breakdown and destabilization of the extracellular matrix.[11] Apart from this, basic fibroblast growth factor (bFGF) is present in the tissues surrounding the injured area and in the tendon sheath and promotes fibroblast proliferation and angiogenesis,[12] which is also known to affect healing after injury. Fibroblast invasion and neovascular vessel formation from the inflammatory response—signaling

molecules such as TGF-β and bFGF—form scar tissue.[13] Fibroblasts and neovascularization within the contours of the tendon contribute to tendon healing; fibroblasts and neovascularization outside the tendon contribute to adhesion formation. Both the healing tendon and adhesions will remodel in response to time and, especially, motion; loading plays a lesser role, beyond the amount of load necessary to induce motion. Beyond that amount, further tendon loading simply increases the risk of rupture, without any further benefit on healing or adhesions.[14] The lubricating components of the tendon surface (HA, phospholipids, and lubricin) may also affect the likelihood and degree of adhesion formation, and early restoration of these components is also an avenue of adhesion prevention research.

OVERVIEW OF METHODS TO PREVENT TENDON ADHESIONS

Research on methods to prevent tendon adhesion formation ranges from early exercise therapy to the introduction of microRNA (miRNA) to alter local gene expression. However, as mentioned above, these methods can be broadly divided into 2 categories: physical barriers to prevent adhesion to the tendon surface and biological treatment to reduce adhesion formation.

Physical Methods

Surgical techniques
Modern surgical techniques can help reduce adhesion formation in 2 ways. First, a stronger repair facilitates early mobilization, and early motion is still the best way to reduce adhesion formation after

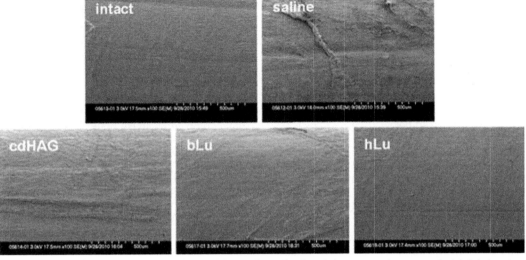

Fig. 2. Scanning electron microscopy images of the surface of palmaris longus tendon treated with lubricants. cd HAG, carbodiimide-derivatized HA and gelatin; bLu, bovine synovial fluid lubricin; hLu, human synoviocyte lubricin. (*Reprinted from* Bio-medical materials and engineering, 21(5-6), Kohn MD, Sun YL, Zhao C, et al., Human synoviocyte lubricin and bovine synovial fluid lubricin equally improve gliding resistance in a canine model in vitro, 281-289, Copyright 2011, with permission from IOS Press. The publication is available at IOS Press through http://dx.doi.org/10.3233/BME-2012-0676.)

tendon injury and repair. Second, the use of less reactive, low-friction suture materials and suture constructs can also reduce friction and gliding resistance of the repair. Repairs that avoid knots on the anterior tendon surface (the side that contacts the pulleys) can reduce abrasion of the tendon surface.[15] Zhao, in their study of canine tendons, showed that single-strand sutures resulted in less adhesion formation compared with multistrand sutures,[16] whereas several reports have found no significant difference between single-strand and multistrand suture methods to adhesion formation after tendon repair.[17,18] Although fewer sutures imply decreased tendon repair strength, it is important to remember the importance of suture caliber to repair strength. A 2-strand repair of 3 to 0 suture is not weaker than 4-strands of 4 to 0 suture, for example.[19]

Repair of tendon sheaths has occasionally been performed and recommended to reduce adhesions.[20] Strauch and Peterson presented reduced adhesion formation with tendon sheath repair in a chicken model.[21,22] However, several other reports have found no significant differences in adhesion formation after sheath repair in human and other animal models.[5,23–25] Most importantly, sheath closure can have a major negative impact on tendon gliding. Thus, contemporary tendon repair methods favor judicious pulley excision to minimize conflict of the tendon repair with overlying pulleys. In zone 1, it is almost always preferable to sacrifice the A4 pulley if there is any

concern about its interference with tendon gliding. Resection of on superficialis slip or a portion of A2 can perform the same function in zone 2 repairs.[26]

Postoperative Mobilization

Postoperative mobilization is the one factor under the surgeon's control that has the greatest impact on decreasing adhesion formation and improving function after tendon repair.[27,28] Numerous postoperative mobilization methods have been proposed,[29–31] ranging from passive to active-assisted to active motion but evidence from randomized controlled trials is insufficient to show the superiority of one method over another, and the best method is still elusive.[2] One thing that does seem clear is that loading, beyond the loading needed to get the tendon to move, does not aid healing or gliding, and may simply risk rupture without a counterbalancing benefit.[32,33]

Biologic Treatments

Hyaluronic acid
Smooth gliding of tendons is achieved by low friction on the tendon surface. This low friction is mainly created by the lubricants HA and lubricin[34] (**Fig. 2**). Many basic studies have been performed in animals with HA administration to injured tendons and have reported good results in improving tendon sliding.[35–37] However, in 1992, Hagberg conducted a prospective, double-blind, randomized clinical trial using 120 fingers, which

unfortunately showed no significant effect of HA treatment.[38] This is likely because the HA is either mechanically cleared or broken down by hyaluronidase within a short time. Subsequent research has focused on increasing the resident time of HA at the repair site to see if that can improve the effectiveness of this treatment.[39,40] Some studies also suggest that HA production may influence adhesion improvement in relation to bFGF signaling, as discussed below.[41]

Lubricin

Lubricin (proteoglycan 4) is a proteoglycan encoded by the *PRG4* gene, discovered in 1981 as a joint-lubricating component produced by articular cartilage.[42–44] In later studies, lubricin has been reported to have not only lubricating effects but also antiadhesive and cytoprotective functions in many tissues.[45] Lubricin is also expressed on the surface of normal tendons, suggesting that this may prevent cell adhesion to the tendon surface. Lubricin synthesis is decreased during tendon inflammation due to injury or disease, suggesting that lubricin downregulation may contribute to tendon adhesion formation.[46,47]

Taguchi and colleagues conducted a study using canine peroneus longus tendons and reported that although lubricin alone did not improve tendon sliding, administration of both lubricin and carbodiimide-derivatized gelatin, combined with HA, significantly improved tendon gliding in vitro.[48] Taguchi also reported that the combined administration of lubricin with carbodiimide-derivatized gelatin and HA significantly improved tendon gliding and reduced adhesion formation in repaired tendons from dogs and cadavers.[49,50] However, Zhao and colleagues conducted a study using an in vivo canine model and reported that the combined administration of lubricin and carbodiimide-derivatized gelatin and HA to repaired tendons, which, although demonstrating a marked reduction in adhesions (**Fig. 3**) and improvement in tendon gliding, also resulted in significantly reduced failure strength of the repaired tendon, suggesting that this treatment may adversely affect tendon healing.[51,52] Subsequent studies adding growth factors and cells under the lubricin and carbodiimide-derivatized gelatin, combined with HA, showed some improvement in healing strength but not up to control levels.

Bioabsorbable Gels

ADCON-T/N (Gliatech, Cleveland, USA), a bioabsorbable gel composed of porcine gelatin, polyglycan esters, and phosphate buffered saline, has been reported to safely reduce perineural scarring[53,54]; Golash and colleagues conducted a prospective, double-blind, randomized study of 50 fingers in which ADCON-T/N was administered after flexor tendon repair.[55] Although ROM was not significantly affected, the time to achieve the final ROM was significantly shorter in the treated group. However, the rate of late rupture was higher in the treated group, suggesting that ADCON-T/N may have inhibited wound healing, similar to the effect of lubricin and carbodiimide-derivatized gelatin combined with HA noted above.

Absorbable Oxidized Regenerated Cellulose

Coating of repaired tendons with absorbable oxidized regenerated cellulose (Interceed, TC-7, Johnson & Johnson, USA) reduced gross and histologic adhesions,[56,57] and the inflammatory response was also reduced.[57] However, these studies were all performed in Achilles tendon models, and the relevance to intrasynovial, sheathed tendons is unknown.

Hydrogels

A polymer of 2-methacryloyloxyethyl phosphorylcholine hydrogels (MPCs) is a type of phospholipid with high biocompatibility.[58] Tendons of rats, chickens, and rabbits were coated with hydrogels containing MPCs, and adhesion formation was reduced without affecting tendon healing. No cytotoxicity was observed.[59,60] MPCs have a honeycomb microstructure with nanometer-sized pores that resist cell invasion but allow the passage of cytokines and growth factors for tendon healing. This particular structure is considered to be responsible for the favorable results. Furthermore, the hydrogel can adjust its degradation rate depending on the concentration of another component, and this study has shown that it can retain its shape for more than 3 weeks, covering the initial essential period in tendon healing.[60]

Hydrogels can also be combined with drugs for more pronounced antiadhesion effects; Karaaltin and colleagues reported that low doses of 5-fluorouracil (5-FU) were filled into hydrogels and released slowly into the repaired tendon area and histologic/biomechanical evaluation showed decreased adhesion formation.[61] Topical 5-FU has been shown to reduce adhesions in animal models and may be useful in cases of tenolysis.[62–64]

Electrospun Fiber Membranes

Electrospun fiber membranes are a method of producing nanofibers using electric fields[65] and can be produced in a variety of forms, including microsols, emulsions, coaxial, and multilayers.[58] They are also biocompatible and have a longer

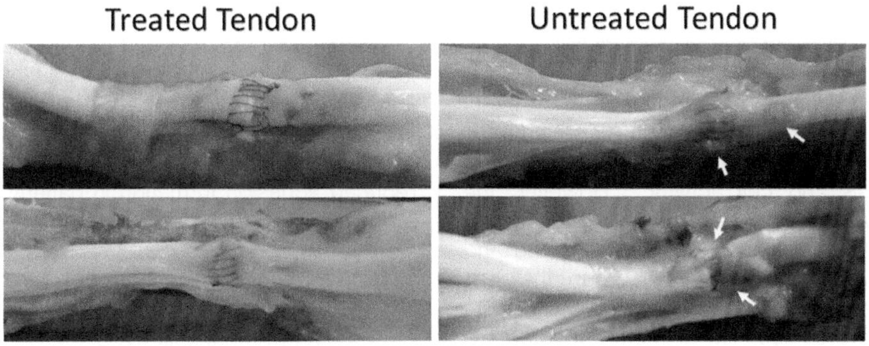

Treated Tendon   Untreated Tendon

Fig. 3. Gross observation of tendons treated by lubricin and carbodiimide-derivatized gelatin and untreated tendons. As observed in the left side panels, treated tendons produced fewer adhesions. (The upper panels present repaired tendons at 21 days posttreatment, and the lower panels present repaired tendons at 42 days posttreatment. The *white arrows* point to adhesions). (*Adapted from* Zhao C, Ozasa Y, Shimura H, et al. Effects of lubricant and autologous bone marrow stromal cell augmentation on immobilized flexor tendon repairs. Journal of Orthopaedic Research : official publication of the Orthopaedic Research Society. 2016;34(1):154-160; with permission.)

degradation time in vivo than hydrogels, making them promising as longer-affecting antiadhesion materials.[65] Furthermore, electrospun fiber membranes have the advantage that they can be used as sustained-release carriers for drugs. However, the role of these products in the intrasynovial environment has not been studied.

CHEMICAL AND MOLECULAR BIOLOGICAL COMPOUND ADDITIONS TO REDUCE SCAR TISSUE FORMATION
Heparin

Heparin is a noncytotoxic, anti-inflammatory agent. It has been suggested that heparin may also affect various stages of tissue repair due to the ability of bFGF to attach to heparin, which plays a vital role in wound healing.[66] Thus, Akbari and colleagues conducted a prospective randomized clinical study of 100 patients with tendon injuries, which showed no improvement in ROM but rather a significantly higher incidence of tendon rupture in heparin-treated tendon repairs.[67]

5-Fluorouracil

5-FU is an anticancer drug with antimetabolic activity but it is said to have antiadhesive properties by inhibiting cell division and cell migration,[68] and in ophthalmology, it was reported to decrease postoperative scar formation.[69,70] Moran and colleagues administered 5-FU to repaired tendons of Leghorn chickens and found a reduction in adhesion formation in histologic evaluation.[63] Others have reported decreased adhesion formation with 5-FU treatment in rabbit in vivo and in vitro models.[62,64,71]

Vitamins C and E

After a tendon injury, the local inflammatory response results in oxidative stress. It has been suggested that reactive oxygen species may play an important role in adhesion formation.[72] Vitamins C and E have been shown to have antagonistic effects on oxidative stress[73,74] and may be useful in preventing adhesion formation.

Repaired chicken tendons treated with vitamin C showed significant improvement in gliding resistance, significant reduction in fibrosis, and histologic examination showed reduced adhesion formation around the tendon.[75] Trolox, a water-soluble analog of vitamin E, administered to repaired chicken tendons showed a similar reduction in fibrosis and adhesions.[76]

Anti-inflammatory Drugs

As mentioned previously, the inflammatory response after a tendon injury is one of the major factors involved in adhesion formation. Various studies have attempted to prevent adhesion formation by suppressing this response. Although in some studies injections and oral administration of ibuprofen and indomethacin have been shown to reduce adhesion formation and improve joint ROM in injured tendons in monkeys and rabbits,[77–80] other studies using oral administration of ibuprofen also showed a decrease in failure strength of repaired tendons.[78]

In recent years, there has also been much research on biomaterials that can contain anti-inflammatory drugs and function as physical barriers.[81]

Basic Fibroblast Growth Factor

bFGF is involved in fibroblast proliferation and angiogenesis, which are also known to strongly affect healing after injury.[12]

Oryan and colleagues reported that administration of bFGF to repaired tendons in rabbits resulted in decreased peritendinous adhesions, collagen production, and maturation and resulted in increased repaired tendon strength.[82] However, Thomopoulos and colleagues administered bFGF to repaired canine tendons and reported the exact opposite: increased tendon adhesion formation and decreased ROM reduction with increased angiogenesis and cell activity.[34] However, the latter study compared the group of bFGF administered to repaired tendons with fibrin-based and heparin-based matrices to the group that just repaired tendon; thus, there is a possibility that the presence or absence of matrix affected the results.

TGF-β/Smad3

As indicated in the introduction, TGF-β is a cytokine strongly associated with adhesion formation and transmits signaling through Smad3.[83] It has been suggested that suppressing TGF-β may prevent tendon adhesions. Chen and colleagues generated miRNA silencing the TGF-β gene, injected it into repaired tendons in chickens and found that in addition to TGF-β, the expression of collagen III and connective tissue growth factor was also reduced.[10] Furthermore, Wu and colleagues transduced TGF-β1-miRNA into repaired tendons of chickens using Adeno-associated virus and obtained improved adhesion scores. However, a 12% to 24% reduction in failure strength was observed in the transduced tendons relative to the control group, simultaneously indicating a possible negative effect on tendon repair.[84]

Other reports include reduced contracture formation in Smad3 knockout mice by suppressing TGF-β signaling[85] and reduced Smad2/3 phosphorylation and adhesion formation by coating repaired tendons with a celecoxib-containing carrier membrane.[86] In the latter, a significant decrease in tendon strength was also demonstrated, presenting the troubling conclusion of reduced adhesion formation and adverse effects on tendon repair due to suppression of TGF-β signaling.

PXL01

PXL01 is a synthetic peptide derived from human lactoferrin, a glycoprotein present in milk and mucosal secretions, which exhibits antibacterial and anti-inflammatory properties.[87,88] When administered to repaired rabbit tendons, lactoferrin significantly improved tendon mobility and had no negative effect on tendon healing strength.[89,90] In addition, Wiig and colleagues conducted a prospective, double-blind, randomized trial in 138 patients.[91] Administration of PXL01 around the repaired tendon resulted in a significant improvement in finger ROM and did not increase

the incidence of tendon rupture. Another molecular biological study has reported that local administration of PXL01 increased the production of lubricin and decreased the production of inflammatory cytokines.[92] These effects may cause reduced adhesion formation in patients' repaired tendons.

Beta Amino Proprionitrile

Beta amino proprionitrile (BAPN) blocks collagen cross-linking and can be effective in reducing adhesions.[93,94] However, its effect is ubiquitous and interferes not only with collagen at the repair site but also at other locations such as arterial walls. Thus, it has not found favor for any clinical use.

SUMMARY

Numerous studies have been conducted using multiple physical and chemical/biologic agents to prevent adhesions, and several methods have presented efficacy at the clinical level. However, many of these methods are accompanied by drawbacks, especially with regard to reducing adhesion formation while maintaining repaired tendon strength, which is unfortunately often a trade-off, and no absolute antiadhesion method has yet been reported to preserve tendon repair strength. In recent years, with the advances in biomaterial science, various polymeric materials that can contain compounds and are both biocompatible and biodegradable have been reported. By using these materials, one may hope that someday reduction of adhesion formation while maintaining repaired tendon strength will no longer be a dream. For now, the best way to reduce adhesions after tendon injury in the hand is to perform a strong, low friction repair, trim pulleys where necessary to allow tendon gliding, and to begin early postoperative rehabilitation when possible.

CLINICS CARE POINTS, PEARLS, AND PITFALLS

- Adhesions are inevitable after tendon injury and worsen with inflammation and neovascularization caused by injury and ischemia.
- The surgeon can reduce adhesions with a strong, low friction repair, judicious pulley trimming, and early mobilization.

- Adhesion barriers and antimetabolites may reduce adhesions in experimental models but currently all come at a cost of delayed healing and increased risk of repair rupture.

DISCLOSURE

The authors have nothing to disclose.

REFERENCES

1. Tang JB. Clinical outcomes associated with flexor tendon repair. Hand Clin 2005;21(2):199–210.
2. Khanna A, Friel M, Gougoulias N, et al. Prevention of adhesions in surgery of the flexor tendons of the hand: what is the evidence? Br Med Bull 2009;90:85–109.
3. Beredjiklian PK. Biologic aspects of flexor tendon laceration and repair. J bone Jt Surg Am volume 2003;85(3):539–50.
4. Amadio PC, Hunter JM, Jaeger SH, et al. The effect of vincular injury on the results of flexor tendon surgery in zone 2. J Hand Surg Am 1985;10(5):626–32.
5. Saldana MJ, Ho PK, Lichtman DM, et al. Flexor tendon repair and rehabilitation in zone II open sheath technique versus closed sheath technique. J Hand Surg Am 1987;12(6):1110–4.
6. Lilly SI, Messer TM. Complications after treatment of flexor tendon injuries. J Am Acad Orthopaedic Surgeons 2006;14(7):387–96.
7. Murray MM, Kalish LA, Fleming BC, et al. Bridge-Enhanced Anterior Cruciate Ligament Repair: Two-Year Results of a First-in-Human Study. Orthopaedic J Sports Med 2019;7(3). 2325967118824356.
8. Chang J, Most D, Stelnicki E, et al. Gene expression of transforming growth factor beta-1 in rabbit zone II flexor tendon wound healing: evidence for dual mechanisms of repair. Plast Reconstr Surg 1997;100(4):937–44.
9. Chang J, Thunder R, Most D, et al. Studies in flexor tendon wound healing: neutralizing antibody to TGF-beta1 increases postoperative range of motion. Plast Reconstr Surg 2000;105(1):148–55.
10. Chen CH, Zhou YL, Wu YF, et al. Effectiveness of microRNA in Down-regulation of TGF-beta gene expression in digital flexor tendons of chickens: in vitro and in vivo study. J Hand Surg Am 2009; 34(10):1777–84. e1771.
11. Maeda T, Sakabe T, Sunaga A, et al. Conversion of mechanical force into TGF-β-mediated biochemical signals. Curr Biol : CB 2011;21(11):933–41.
12. Chang J, Most D, Thunder R, et al. Molecular studies in flexor tendon wound healing: the role of basic fibroblast growth factor gene expression. J Hand Surg Am 1998;23(6):1052–8.
13. Whitby DJ, Ferguson MW. Immunohistochemical localization of growth factors in fetal wound healing. Developmental Biol 1991;147(1):207–15.
14. Boyer MI, Gelberman RH, Burns ME, et al. Intrasynovial flexor tendon repair. An experimental study comparing low and high levels of in vivo force during rehabilitation in canines. J bone Jt Surg Am volume 2001;83(6):891–9.
15. Elliot D, Giesen T. Primary flexor tendon surgery: the search for a perfect result. Hand Clin 2013;29(2): 191–206.
16. Zhao C, Amadio PC, Momose T, et al. The effect of suture technique on adhesion formation after flexor tendon repair for partial lacerations in a canine model. J Trauma 2001;51(5):917–21.
17. Strick MJ, Filan SL, Hile M, et al. Adhesion formation after flexor tendon repair: a histologic and biomechanical comparison of 2- and 4-strand repairs in a chicken model. J Hand Surg Am 2004;29(1): 15–21.
18. Thurman RT, Trumble TE, Hanel DP, et al. Two-, four-, and six-strand zone II flexor tendon repairs: an in situ biomechanical comparison using a cadaver model. J Hand Surg Am 1998;23(2):261–5.
19. Barrie KA, Tomak SL, Cholewicki J, et al. Effect of suture locking and suture caliber on fatigue strength of flexor tendon repairs. J Hand Surg Am 2001;26(2): 340–6.
20. Matthews P, Richards H. The repair potential of digital flexor tendons. An experimental study. J bone Jt Surg Br 1974;56-b(4):618–25.
21. Peterson WW, Manske PR, Dunlap J, et al. Effect of various methods of restoring flexor sheath integrity on the formation of adhesions after tendon injury. J Hand Surg Am 1990;15(1):48–56.
22. Strauch B, de Moura W, Ferder M, et al. The fate of tendon healing after restoration of the integrity of the tendon sheath with autogenous vein grafts. J Hand Surg Am 1985;10(6 Pt 1):790–5.
23. Gelberman RH, Woo SL, Amiel D, et al. Influences of flexor sheath continuity and early motion on tendon healing in dogs. J Hand Surg Am 1990;15(1):69–77.
24. Peterson WW, Manske PR, Kain CC, et al. Effect of flexor sheath integrity on tendon gliding: a biomechanical and histologic study. J orthopaedic Res 1986;4(4):458–65.
25. Tang JB. Flexor tendon repair in zone 2C. J Hand Surg (Edinburgh, Scotland) 1994;19(1):72–5.
26. Paillard PJ, Amadio PC, Zhao C, et al. Pulley plasty versus resection of one slip of the flexor digitorum superficialis after repair of both flexor tendons in zone II: a biomechanical study. J bone Jt Surg Am volume 2002;84(11):2039–45.
27. Strickland JW, Glogovac SV. Digital function following flexor tendon repair in Zone II: A comparison of immobilization and controlled passive motion techniques. J Hand Surg Am 1980;5(6):537–43.

28. Wilson K, Moore MJ, Rayner CR, et al. Extensor tendon repair: an animal model which allows immediate post-operative mobilisation. J Hand Surg (Edinburgh, Scotland) 1990;15(1):74–8.

29. Gelberman RH, Nunley JA 2nd, Osterman AL, et al. Influences of the protected passive mobilization interval on flexor tendon healing. A prospective randomized clinical study. Clin Orthop Relat Res 1991;(264):189–96.

30. Percival NJ, Sykes PJ. Flexor pollicis longus tendon repair: a comparison between dynamic and static splintage. J Hand Surg (Edinburgh, Scotland) 1989;14(4):412–5.

31. Tang JB, Ishii S, Usui M, et al. Flexor sheath closure during delayed primary tendon repair. J Hand Surg Am 1994;19(4):636–40.

32. Dinopoulos HT, Boyer MI, Burns ME, et al. The resistance of a four- and eight-strand suture technique to gap formation during tensile testing: an experimental study of repaired canine flexor tendons after 10 days of in vivo healing. J Hand Surg Am 2000;25(3):489–98.

33. Nessler JP, Amadio PC, Berglund LJ, et al. Healing of canine tendon in zones subjected to different mechanical forces. J Hand Surg (Edinburgh, Scotland) 1992;17(5):561–8.

34. Thomopoulos S, Kim HM, Das R, et al. The effects of exogenous basic fibroblast growth factor on intrasynovial flexor tendon healing in a canine model. J bone Jt Surg Am volume 2010;92(13):2285–93.

35. Rydell N, Balazs EA. Effect of intra-articular injection of hyaluronic acid on the clinical symptoms of osteoarthritis and on granulation tissue formation. Clin Orthop Relat Res 1971;80:25–32.

36. St Onge R, Weiss C, Denlinger JL, et al. A preliminary assessment of Na-hyaluronate injection into "no man's land" for primary flexor tendon repair. Clin Orthop Relat Res 1980;(146):269–75.

37. Uchiyama S, Amadio PC, Ishikawa J, et al. Boundary lubrication between the tendon and the pulley in the finger. J bone Jt Surg Am volume 1997;79(2):213–8.

38. Hagberg L. Exogenous hyaluronate as an adjunct in the prevention of adhesions after flexor tendon surgery: a controlled clinical trial. J Hand Surg Am 1992;17(1):132–6.

39. Momose T, Amadio PC, Sun YL, et al. Surface modification of extrasynovial tendon by chemically modified hyaluronic acid coating. J Biomed Mater Res 2002;59(2):219–24.

40. Yang C, Amadio PC, Sun YL, et al. Tendon surface modification by chemically modified HA coating after flexor digitorum profundus tendon repair. J Biomed Mater Res B, Appl Biomater 2004;68(1):15–20.

41. Thomopoulos S, Das R, Sakiyama-Elbert S, et al. bFGF and PDGF-BB for tendon repair: controlled release and biologic activity by tendon fibroblasts in vitro. Ann Biomed Eng 2010;38(2):225–34.

42. Schumacher BL, Block JA, Schmid TM, et al. A novel proteoglycan synthesized and secreted by chondrocytes of the superficial zone of articular cartilage. Arch Biochem Biophys 1994;311(1):144–52.

43. Swann DA, Silver FH, Slayter HS, et al. The molecular structure and lubricating activity of lubricin isolated from bovine and human synovial fluids. Biochem J 1985;225(1):195–201.

44. Swann DA, Slayter HS, Silver FH. The molecular structure of lubricating glycoprotein-I, the boundary lubricant for articular cartilage. J Biol Chem 1981;256(11):5921–5.

45. Sun Y, Berger EJ, Zhao C, et al. Mapping lubricin in canine musculoskeletal tissues. Connect Tissue Res 2006;47(4):215–21.

46. Rees SG, Davies JR, Tudor D, et al. Immunolocalisation and expression of proteoglycan 4 (cartilage superficial zone proteoglycan) in tendon. Matrix Biol : J Int Soc Matrix Biol 2002;21(7):593–602.

47. Sun YL, Zhao C, Jay GD, et al. Effects of stress deprivation on lubricin synthesis and gliding of flexor tendons in a canine model in vivo. J bone Jt Surg Am volume 2013;95(3):273–8.

48. Taguchi M, Sun YL, Zhao C, et al. Lubricin surface modification improves extrasynovial tendon gliding in a canine model in vitro. J bone Jt Surg Am volume 2008;90(1):129–35.

49. Taguchi M, Sun YL, Zhao C, et al. Lubricin surface modification improves tendon gliding after tendon repair in a canine model in vitro. J orthopaedic Res 2009;27(2):257–63.

50. Taguchi M, Zhao C, Sun YL, et al. The effect of surface treatment using hyaluronic acid and lubricin on the gliding resistance of human extrasynovial tendons in vitro. J Hand Surg Am 2009;34(7):1276–81.

51. Zhao C, Hashimoto T, Kirk RL, et al. Resurfacing with chemically modified hyaluronic acid and lubricin for flexor tendon reconstruction. J orthopaedic Res 2013;31(6):969–75.

52. Zhao C, Ozasa Y, Shimura H, et al. Effects of lubricant and autologous bone marrow stromal cell augmentation on immobilized flexor tendon repairs. J orthopaedic Res 2016;34(1):154–60.

53. Palatinsky EA, Maier KH, Touhalisky DK, et al. ADCON-T/N reduces in vivo perineural adhesions in a rat sciatic nerve reoperation model. J Hand Surg (Edinburgh, Scotland) 1997;22(3):331–5.

54. Petersen J, Russell L, Andrus K, et al. Reduction of extraneural scarring by ADCON-T/N after surgical intervention. Neurosurgery 1996;38(5):976–83 [discussion: 983-974].

55. Golash A, Kay A, Warner JG, et al. Efficacy of ADCON-T/N after primary flexor tendon repair in Zone II: a controlled clinical trial. J Hand Surg (Edinburgh, Scotland) 2003;28(2):113–5.

56. Meislin RJ, Wiseman DM, Alexander H, et al. A biomechanical study of tendon adhesion reduction using a biodegradable barrier in a rabbit model. J Appl Biomater : official J Soc Biomater 1990;1(1): 13–9.

57. Temiz A, Ozturk C, Bakunov A, et al. A new material for prevention of peritendinous fibrotic adhesions after tendon repair: oxidised regenerated cellulose (Interceed), an absorbable adhesion barrier. Int orthopaedics 2008;32(3):389–94.

58. Zhou H, Lu H. Advances in the Development of Anti-Adhesive Biomaterials for Tendon Repair Treatment. Tissue Eng regenerative Med 2021;18(1):1–14.

59. Ishiyama N, Moro T, Ishihara K, et al. The prevention of peritendinous adhesions by a phospholipid polymer hydrogel formed in situ by spontaneous intermolecular interactions. Biomaterials 2010;31(14): 4009–16.

60. Ishiyama N, Moro T, Ohe T, et al. Reduction of Peritendinous adhesions by hydrogel containing biocompatible phospholipid polymer MPC for tendon repair. J bone Jt Surg Am volume 2011; 93(2):142–9.

61. Karaaltin MV, Ozalp B, Dadaci M, et al. The effects of 5-fluorouracil on flexor tendon healing by using a biodegradable gelatin, slow releasing system: experimental study in a hen model. J Hand Surg Eur 2013;38(6):651–7.

62. Akali A, Khan U, Khaw PT, et al. Decrease in adhesion formation by a single application of 5-fluorouracil after flexor tendon injury. Plast Reconstr Surg 1999;103(1):151–8.

63. Moran SL, Ryan CK, Orlando GS, et al. Effects of 5-fluorouracil on flexor tendon repair. J Hand Surg Am 2000;25(2):242–51.

64. Ragoowansi R, Khan U, Brown RA, et al. Reduction in matrix metalloproteinase production by tendon and synovial fibroblasts after a single exposure to 5-fluorouracil. Br J Plast Surg 2001;54(4):283–7.

65. Wu W, Cheng R, das Neves J, et al. Advances in biomaterials for preventing tissue adhesion. J controlled release : official J Controlled Release Soc 2017;261:318–36.

66. Zakrzewska M, Wiedlocha A, Szlachcic A, et al. Increased protein stability of FGF1 can compensate for its reduced affinity for heparin. J Biol Chem 2009; 284(37):25388–403.

67. Akbari H, Rahimi AA, Ghavami Y, et al. Effect of Heparin on Post-Operative Adhesion in Flexor Tendon Surgery of the Hand. J Hand microsurgery 2015; 7(2):244–9.

68. Legrand A, Kaufman Y, Long C, et al. Molecular Biology of Flexor Tendon Healing in Relation to Reduction of Tendon Adhesions. J Hand Surg Am 2017;42(9):722–6.

69. Cerovac S, Afoke A, Akali A, et al. Early breaking strength of repaired flexor tendon treated with 5-fluorouracil. J Hand Surg (Edinburgh, Scotland) 2001;26(3):220–3.

70. Khaw PT, Occleston NL, Schultz G, et al. Activation and suppression of fibroblast function. Eye (London, England) 1994;8(Pt 2):188–95.

71. Duci SB, Arifi HM, Ahmeti HR, et al. Biomechanical and Macroscopic Evaluations of the Effects of 5-Fluorouracil on Partially Divided Flexor Tendon Injuries in Rabbits. Chin Med J 2015;128(12): 1655–61.

72. Binda MM, Molinas CR, Koninckx PR. Reactive oxygen species and adhesion formation: clinical implications in adhesion prevention. Hum Reprod (Oxford, England) 2003;18(12):2503–7.

73. Padayatty SJ, Katz A, Wang Y, et al. Vitamin C as an antioxidant: evaluation of its role in disease prevention. J Am Coll Nutr 2003;22(1):18–35.

74. Traber MG, Atkinson J. Vitamin E, antioxidant and nothing more. Free Radic Biol Med 2007;43(1):4–15.

75. Hung LK, Fu SC, Lee YW, et al. Local vitamin-C injection reduced tendon adhesion in a chicken model of flexor digitorum profundus tendon injury. J bone Jt Surg Am volume 2013;95(7):e41.

76. Lee YW, Fu SC, Mok TY, et al. Local administration of Trolox, a vitamin E analog, reduced tendon adhesion in a chicken model of flexor digitorum profundus tendon injury. J orthopaedic translation 2017;10: 102–7.

77. Kulick MI, Brazlow R, Smith S, et al. Injectable ibuprofen: preliminary evaluation of its ability to decrease peritendinous adhesions. Ann Plast Surg 1984;13(6):459–67.

78. Kulick MI, Smith S, Hadler K. Oral ibuprofen: evaluation of its effect on peritendinous adhesions and the breaking strength of a tenorrhaphy. J Hand Surg Am 1986;11(1):110–20.

79. Szabo RM, Younger E. Effects of indomethacin on adhesion formation after repair of zone II tendon lacerations in the rabbit. J Hand Surg Am 1990;15(3): 480–3.

80. Tan V, Nourbakhsh A, Capo J, et al. Effects of nonsteroidal anti-inflammatory drugs on flexor tendon adhesion. J Hand Surg Am 2010;35(6): 941–7.

81. Brebels J, Mignon A. Polymer-Based Constructs for Flexor Tendon Repair: A Review. Polymers 2022; 14(5).

82. Oryan A, Moshiri A. Recombinant fibroblast growth protein enhances healing ability of experimentally induced tendon injury in vivo. J Tissue Eng regenerative Med 2014;8(6):421–31.

83. Jiang K, Chun G, Wang Z, et al. Effect of transforming growth factor-β3 on the expression of Smad3 and Smad7 in tenocytes. Mol Med Rep 2016;13(4): 3567–73.

84. Wu YF, Mao WF, Zhou YL, et al. Adeno-associated virus-2-mediated TGF-β1 microRNA transfection

inhibits adhesion formation after digital flexor tendon injury. Gene Ther 2016;23(2):167–75.

85. Katzel EB, Koltz PF, Tierney R, et al. The impact of Smad3 loss of function on TGF-β signaling and radiation-induced capsular contracture. Plast Reconstr Surg 2011;127(6):2263–9.

86. Jiang S, Zhao X, Chen S, et al. Down-regulating ERK1/2 and SMAD2/3 phosphorylation by physical barrier of celecoxib-loaded electrospun fibrous membranes prevents tendon adhesions. Biomaterials 2014;35(37):9920–9.

87. Legrand D, Elass E, Pierce A, et al. Lactoferrin and host defence: an overview of its immunomodulating and anti-inflammatory properties. Biometals : Int J role metal ions Biol Biochem Med 2004;17(3):225–9.

88. Ward PP, Uribe-Luna S, Conneely OM. Lactoferrin and host defense. Biochem Cel Biol = Biochimie biologie cellulaire 2002;80(1):95–102.

89. Håkansson J, Mahlapuu M, Ekström L, et al. Effect of lactoferrin peptide (PXL01) on rabbit digit mobility after flexor tendon repair. J Hand Surg Am 2012; 37(12):2519–25.

90. Wiig M, Olmarker K, Håkansson J, et al. A lactoferrin-derived peptide (PXL01) for the reduction of adhesion formation in flexor tendon surgery: an experimental study in rabbits. J Hand Surg Eur volume 2011;36(8):656–62.

91. Wiig ME, Dahlin LB, Fridén J, et al. PXL01 in sodium hyaluronate for improvement of hand recovery after flexor tendon repair surgery: randomized controlled trial. PloS one 2014;9(10):e110735.

92. Edsfeldt S, Holm B, Mahlapuu M, et al. PXL01 in sodium hyaluronate results in increased PRG4 expression: a potential mechanism for anti-adhesion. Upsala J Med Sci 2017;122(1):28–34.

93. Furlow LT Jr, Peacock EE Jr. Effect of beta-amino propionitrile on the prevention and treatment of joint stiffness in rats. Surg Forum 1965;16:457–8.

94. Smiley JD, Yeager H, Ziff M. Collagen metabolism in osteolathyrism in chick embryos: site of action of beta-amino-propionitrile. J Exp Med 1962;116(1): 45–54.

Therapy after Flexor Tendon Repair

Terri M. Skirven, BScOT, OTR/L, CHT*, Lauren M. DeTullio, MOT, OTR/L, CHT

KEYWORDS

- Early motion • Dorsal protective orthosis • Tendon gliding • Tendon protocol • Place-hold
- Excursion • Adhesions • Passive motion

KEY POINTS

- The goal of therapy after flexor tendon repair is the early restoration of tendon gliding and prevention of restrictive adhesion formation while protecting the repair from rupture and the maintenance or restoration of digital joint mobility.
- The selection of a postoperative protocol after flexor tendon repair whether passive, active, or active/passive is based on the surgical procedure performed and the surgeon's assessment of the capacity of the repair to withstand the forces imparted to the tendon during motion; as well as the patient's ability to understand and follow directions and be compliant with the home program instructions and precautions.
- Tendon protocols are meant to serve as guidelines for postoperative management and not as rigid timetables for when different exercises may be introduced. Rather, clinical judgment and reasoning must be used to advance a patient's therapy program and should be based on patient's progress or lack of progress.
- Immoderate tendon loading with exercises and use risks tendon rupture and therefore progression of the therapy program after flexor tendon repair must be done with care and collaboration between the surgeon and therapist.
- A not uncommon problem encountered after flexor tendon repair during the rehabilitation process is flexion contracture of the PIP joint of the involved digit. The first and best approach is prevention of contractures by careful orthosis fabrication and positioning of the involved digit. Ongoing monitoring of the fit of the dorsal block orthosis at each therapy visit is essential to prevent the loss of appropriate positioning from the reduction in edema and dressings.

INTRODUCTION

Rehabilitation after flexor tendon repair has evolved during the last several decades and has been based on the evolving understanding of tendon nutrition and healing and the factors that influence it. These factors include the development of suture repair techniques, the response of the tendon to applied stress (motion), and prompted by the goal of improved and consistent outcomes. This evolution is reflected in the progression in clinical practice from initial immobilization of repaired tendons to early controlled passive motion to the current practice of early active motion combined with passive. Numerous protocols have been developed with variations in patterns of motion, timing, and orthosis designs and positions. The common goal of all of the protocols is the early restoration of tendon gliding while protecting the repair from rupture and the maintenance or restoration of digital joint mobility.

The authors have nothing to disclose.
Philadelphia Hand to Shoulder Center, Therapy Department, 950 Pulaski Drive, Suite 100, King of Prussia, PA 19406, USA
* Corresponding author. 950 Pulaski Drive, Suite 100, King of Prussia, PA 19406.
E-mail address: tskirven@handcenters.com

hand.theclinics.com

HISTORICAL PERSPECTIVE

Mason and Allen's experiments in 1941[1] supported the practice of initial immobilization of repaired flexor tendons. In their studies of the rate at which a repaired tendon regains its tensile strength in a canine model, Mason and Allen reported 2 significant findings. First, there was a profound decrease in tensile strength of the tendon repair with the lowest values measured 4 to 5 days after repair. The tendon stumps had little holding power, and the suture pulled out of the tendon when stress was applied. Although tensile strength gradually increased for up to 10 days, the repair was considered incapable of responding to externally applied stress during this time. The second finding was that, after 19 days, the tensile strength of the repair increased directly with the stresses applied to it. These findings influenced clinicians to immobilize repaired tendons for 3 weeks before allowing attempts at active tendon gliding.

Potenza's research reported in 1963[2] also supported the practice of initial immobilization of flexor tendon repairs. In a canine model, he studied the healing response of repaired tendons that were encased in a synthetic tube to block the ingrowth of adhesions. He found necrosis of the tendon repair at 32 days after repair, with no intrinsic healing activity observed in the tendon itself, and thought that the degeneration of the tendon within the tube represented an avascular phenomenon. Potenza concluded that no intrinsic fibroblastic response from the injured tissue occurred and that healing depends on extrinsic cellular ingrowth. Rather than prevent adhesions, Potenza concluded that adhesions were necessary and should be allowed to form without disruption, thus supporting the concept of immobilization during the early weeks following flexor tendon repair.

Peacock in 1965[3] subsequently proposed the "one wound concept," which supported the extrinsic healing theory. The "one wound concept" refers to the fact that the early process of wound healing is the same in all tissues involved in the injury. During the first stage of healing—the inflammatory stage—the tendon wound site is filled uniformly with leukocytes, macrophages, fluids, and other inflammatory elements, which leave the vascular system. During the second stage of proliferation or fibroplasia, fibroblasts synthesize and extrude collagen. Peacock stated that the fibroblasts migrated from adjacent areas and that the tendon itself did not contain many cells capable of synthesizing collagen. Initially, the collagen is in a random network that links all parts of the wound. It is during the next phase of remodeling that differentiation of healing between different parts of the wound occurs. With a successful repair, the collagen between the tendon ends becomes reoriented into polarized parallel bundles that have great strength similar to normal tendon, whereas the collagen between the tendon and adjacent tissues remains elastic and mobile and randomly oriented.[4]

What factors influence this remodeling and differentiation? Peacock[3] found that the amount of trauma and subsequent tissue damage was related to the extent of remodeling. The lesser the trauma, the more successful and complete the remodeling. Moreover, he thought that newly synthesized scar remodels in response to inductive influences of the tissue with which it is in intimate contact. Other factors relevant to postoperative management are motion and stress. Longitudinal stress and shearing force transmitted by muscle pull along a repaired tendon provokes polarization of the collagen fibers and hence promotes developing strength.[4] The reality, however, is that scar remodeling following initial immobilization of a repaired flexor tendon is not a predictable process and that tendon adherence with some limitation of motion invariably results. The desire to improve the functional outcome of flexor tendon repairs led to the investigation of alternative mechanisms of healing.

Because the response of the tendon to injury depends on its nutrition, the next focus of investigation was on defining more precisely the nutrient pathway to the flexor tendon within the sheath. The tendon passes freely through the sheath with attachment solely by 2 narrow bands of tissue known as vincula. Early investigators thought that these provided a mechanical supporting function but ultimately recognized the vincula as the vascular line to the tendon. Vascular injection studies revealed an intricate intratendinous network derived from 3 sources: the vinculum longum, vinculum brevi, and longitudinal palmar vessels.[5] These studies showed that the intratendinous vessels are located on the dorsum of the tendon and that there are significant areas of avascularity on the volar surface of the tendon and in the zones of the pulleys. These studies led some to conclude that a cooperative system of nutrition, including the intrinsic vasculature and the synovial fluid, was involved in nourishing the tendon.

Manske and colleagues,[6,7] in the late 1970s, in a series of experiments found that the process of synovial fluid diffusion functioned more quickly and completely than did perfusion and was a relatively more important pathway for nutrition.

About the same time, based on their studies, Lundborg and Rank[8] concluded that an intrinsic healing potential existed with nutrition supplied by synovial fluid.

With the existence of an intrinsic healing potential fueled by a synovial fluid nutrient pathway established, studies turned to those factors thought to promote intrinsic healing. Because immobilization supports adhesion formation, investigations turned to the effects of early motion following tendon repairs. Gelberman and colleagues[9] (1980–1982) studied the effects of motion on the healing of canine flexor tendons compared with immobilization and found that the tendons treated with early motion showed higher tensile strength and improved gliding function over the immobilized tendons at each postoperative interval assessed. Early motion stimulated a reorientation of blood vessels to a more normal pattern, whereas immobilization beyond 3 weeks resulted in a random vascular pattern. DNA content was assessed as an indicator of tissue cellularity and repair activity. The tendons that were treated with motion showed a significant increase in DNA, whereas the immobilized tendons were not altered. Gelberman and colleagues[10] also found an absence of adhesion formation and restoration of a gliding surface with the early motion group compared with the dense adhesions seen with the immobilized tendons, which obliterated the space between the tendon and the sheath. They concluded that early motion was the trigger for stimulating an intrinsic repair process and would yield better results than initial immobilization.

The concept of early motion was not a new one. In the 1970s, Kleinert[11] and Duran[12] advocated early controlled motion as a means of producing less restrictive adhesions and thus resulting in better tendon glide. Both techniques initiated passive flexion and blocked extension, with Kleinert advocating active extension (**Fig. 1**, A, B) and Duran and colleagues describing passive extension (**Fig. 2**, A–C). Later investigators described passive programs that incorporated elements of both approaches such as the Washington regimen.[13] These protocols and modifications will be discussed in more detail later in the article.

Clinical studies[14] comparing early passive motion with immobilization found that tendons treated with early motion had a greater average total active motion (TAM) and a greater percentage of excellent results when compared with tendon treated with immobilization. However, the technique of early controlled motion was not without complications and results were not consistently good. Kessler[15] and others questioned whether passive motion produced any significant tendon

motion at all. The suture site may not glide proximally during passive flexion; rather the segment of the tendon distal to the repair site may kink or buckle during passive flexion and then be stretched during limited active extension. Kessler[15] pointed out that gliding of the suture site takes place only by *active* flexion of the operated digit, thus pointing the way toward the development of suture techniques capable of withstanding the forces imparted to the tendon, with active motion combined with the development of orthotic fabrication and controlled active motion protocols. Early examples of these active motion protocols include those of Strickland and Cannon,[16] Silverskiold and May,[17] and Evans and Thompson.[18] Relatively more recent protocols include the Saint John protocol,[19] the Nantong protocol,[20] the Manchester Motion protocol,[21] and a Relative Motion program for zone I/II flexor digitorum profundus (FDP) repairs.[22]

PHASES OF REHABILITATION

Postoperative rehabilitation for flexor tendon repairs is generally guided by the stages of wound healing and can be conceptualized in phases. Phase one can be termed the Protective Phase from 0 to 4 weeks when the strength of the repair is basically that of the suture and any motion program must observe the tensile limits of the repair. Any scar tissue that has formed is weak and easily disrupted by force. The transitional phase is from 4 to 6 weeks when repair strength increases with the beginning of scar tissue maturation and the tensile demands on the repair can be increased but caution must still be observed so as not to disrupt the repair. The extent of scar formation is assessed at this point by the initial tendon excursion. The better the excursion at this phase, the more the tendon is protected from excessive force because adhesion formation is assumed to be minimal, and the tendon may be at a greater risk of rupture. The third phase is full mobilization, which generally begins at 6 weeks and is gradually increased over time as the repair increases in tensile strength. A Pyramid of Progressive Force application has been introduced by Groth[23] and is useful as a clinical reasoning tool to determine when and how to progress motion programs for individual patients.

CLINICAL EVALUATION

Following tendon repair and rehabilitation, total active motion (TAM) and total passive motion (TPM) measurements are used to assess outcome. TAM is calculated by adding the

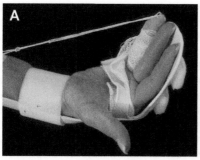
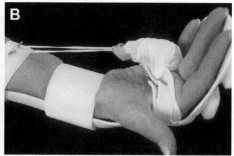

Fig. 1. (*A, B*) *Kleinert program* of controlled passive motion. (*A*) Active extension against the resistance of the elastic band (*B*) with a passive pull back to flexion.

measurement of metacarpophalangeal (MCP), proximal interphalangeal (PIP), and distal interphalangeal (DIP) joint flexion in a fisted position and subtracting the sum of extension deficits at these joints. Strickland[24] advocates a formula, which omits the measurement at the MCP joint. TAM is calculated using only the measurements at the PIP and DIP joints and is divided by 175 multiplied by 100 to give the percentage of normal PIP and DIP motion. A score of 175 represents the normal TAM of these joints in most individuals.

Strickland [24] grades flexor tendon repairs from poor to excellent based on the return of normal motion. Excellent means 75% to 100% of return; good means 50% to 74% of return; fair equals 25% to 49% of return; and poor is 0 to 24% of return.

APPROACHES AND PROTOCOLS

Early motion programs involve controlled motion of the tendon repair starting within the first week and continuing until 3 to 4 weeks postoperatively. Early motion programs require patients who can follow directions, attend therapy, and are reliable; a knowledgeable therapist (ideally a certified hand therapist); and no concomitant injuries precluding early motion. Programs involve passive, active, or synergistic motion and relative motion programs for FDP repairs zone I/II.

Active motion—Widely used, these programs begin at 3 to 5 days after surgery and involve a light active flexor muscle contraction, through either a place and hold partial or full fist, or with "true active motion" with a half a fist. It is important to note that active programs require a suture technique capable of withstanding the forces imparted to the tendon with active motion—usually a strong multistrand core suture method with a simpler peripheral suture.[25] Representative protocols include the following:

Nantong protocol[25] (*Jin Bo Tang*): A combined passive–active motion starts at 4 to 6 days postoperatively. The wrist is positioned in the orthosis at neutral with the hand in a resting position. Partial midrange active finger flexion is preceded by passive finger flexion/extension and is allowed in the first few weeks after surgery (**Fig. 3** A, B). Before attempting active motion, full passive finger flexion and extension exercises—10 to 30 repetitions—are incorporated for patients with edema and/or stiffness to lessen resistance encountered by the repaired tendon with active motion efforts. Starting in weeks 4 to 5 a full range of active finger flexion is allowed and the orthosis is discontinued after week 6.

Saint John *Protocol*:[19] This program calls for combined passive–active motion at 3 to 5 days after surgery. A dorsal block orthosis (DBO) is used with the wrist in 45° extension, the MCP joints in 30° flexion, and the interphalangeal (IP) joints in full extension. Exercises include passive motion of all digits; full IPJ extension with the MCP in full

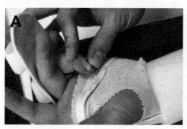
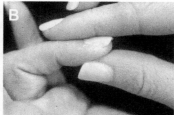
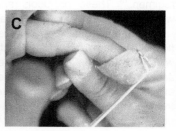

Fig. 2. (*A–C*). *Duran technique* to prevent cross union between the repaired FDS and FDP. (*A*) Passive PIP, DIP flexion; (*B*) passive DIP extension with MCP and PIP flexed glides the FDP suture site away from the FDS suture site; and (*C*) passive PIP extension with the MCP and DIP flexed glides both suture sites away from the site of injury.

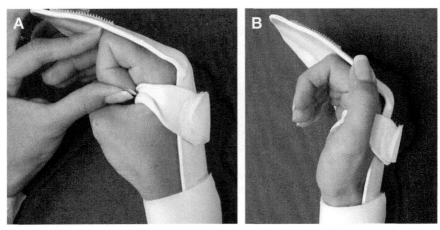

Fig. 3. (*A*, *B*) *Nantong program*–combined passive and active program. (*A*) First, full digit passive flexion and extension within the dorsal protective orthosis to lessen resistance encountered by the repaired tendon with active motion efforts; (*B*) active extension and partial midrange active finger flexion until weeks 4 to 5 at which time a full-range active finger flexion is allowed.

flexion; true active flexion (not place-hold) up to one-third to one-half a fist (active hook fist). At 2 to 4 weeks after surgery, the DBO is shortened as in the Manchester Short Splint (**Fig. 4**). Active synergistic exercise is performed in the short orthosis. Active motion is advanced from half to a full active fist by 6 weeks. Full IP extension is allowed with MCPs in full flexion. At 6 weeks, the orthosis is discontinued.

Manchester Program:[21] This program initiates combined passive/active motion on the fourth to fifth postoperative day. The Manchester Short orthosis extends from the proximal wrist crease to the fingertips and permits full wrist flexion and up to 45° extension with a block of 30° MCP joint extension (**Fig. 4 A–D**). Full passive IP joint flexion exercises precede active motion exercises. Digital flexion exercises are performed in the orthosis; finger extension is

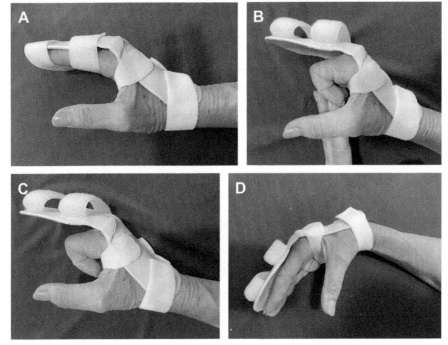

Fig. 4. (*A–D*) *Manchester program* (*A*) short orthosis allows full wrist flexion and 45° wrist extension: (*B*) Full passive IP joint exercises precede (*C*) active flexion performed in the Manchester orthosis with the wrist at the 45° allowed by the orthosis. (*D*) Finger extension with wrist flexed.

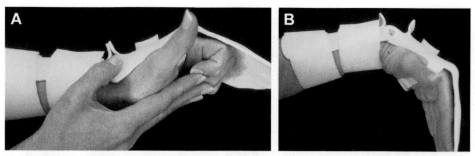

Fig. 5. (*A, B*) *Indiana program hinged wrist orthosis.* (*A*) The patient passively flexes the digits and actively extends the wrist to the 30° allowed by the orthosis with the MCP joints positioned at 45° to 60° of flexion; the patient then lightly holds the digits in the flexed posture. (*B*). Next the patient relaxes and allows the wrist to fall into flexion with the digits extending to the limits of the orthosis through tenodesis effect.

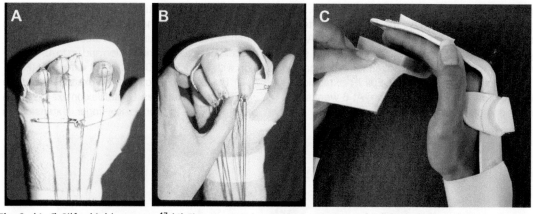

Fig. 6. (*A–C*) *Silferskiold program.*[17] (*A*) Finger extension against resistance of 4-finger elastic traction pulled to a volar attachment point. All 4 fingers are included; (*B*) fingers relax and are pulled back to a flexed position by the elastic traction with further manual passive flexion of the digits; With the passive flexion maintained, the patient attempts an active hold. No unassisted active flexion hold is allowed. (*C*) Elastic traction is released at night with Velcro strap in place to prevent flexion contractures from developing.

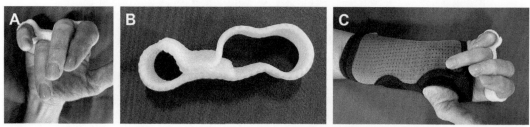

Fig. 7. (*A–C*) *RMF orthoses (RMFO) for zone I, II flexor tendon repairs.*[22] (*A*) RMFO positions the ring MCP joint in 30° to 40° flexion relative to the adjacent MCP joints; (*B*) close-up of RMFO; and (*C*) RMFO worn with a static prefabricated wrist orthosis with wrist at 0° to 20° of wrist extension.

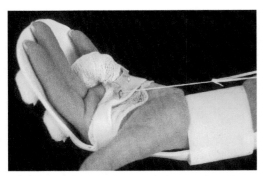

Fig. 8. *Washington regimen* combines the Kleinert and Duran program with the addition of a palmar pulley to increase DIP flexion/FDP excursion.

performed with the wrist flexed. Orthosis use continues until 6 weeks postoperatively.

Indiana Program:[16] This program incorporates 2 orthoses: a dorsal static protective orthosis with wrist at 15° to 30° extension, MCP joints at 45° of flexion and IP joints in extension; and a hinged wrist orthosis, which is worn during an active place and hold exercise. The hinged orthosis allows 30° of wrist extension and positions the MCP joints between 45° and 60° of flexion. Within the orthosis passive placement of the digits in a composite fist position is followed by passively extending the wrist. The patient then actively holds the fisted position. This is followed by relaxing the hand and allowing the wrist to drop into flexion (**Fig. 5**A, B). Exercises are advanced at 4 to 6 weeks.

Silfverskiold Program:[17] This program allows active extension and passive/active flexion. The DBO with wrist neutral and the MCP joints blocked at 60° is used. Elastic traction is attached to all digits pulled through a palmar pulley and secured to a proximal attachment point. Patient performs active extension against the resistance of the elastics within the orthosis; patient then relaxes allowing passive pull back into flexion by the elastics followed by further manual passive flexion to the distal palmar crease. The patient then attempts to hold the digits flexed with the simultaneous flexion positioning by the elastics (place and active assisted hold). The program is progressed after 4 weeks with unassisted active flexion and extension exercises (**Fig. 6** A–C).

Relative Motion:[22] A retrospective case series was published of FDP 4 strand repairs in zone I/II using a relative motion flexion (RMF) orthosis for 8 to 10 weeks in combination with a static dorsal blocking orthosis for the initial 3 weeks. The RMF orthosis positioned the involved digits MCP joint in 30° to 40° of flexion relative to the adjacent MCP joints (**Fig. 7** A–C). The DBO positioned the wrist at 0° to 20° of flexion. Both orthoses were used full time for the first 3 weeks. Exercises included passive composite IP joint flexion and active IP joint extension exercises to neutral with MCP joints flexed, and active finger motion in the RMF orthosis. At 3 weeks, the RMF orthosis continued full time and the DBO was worn at night and for selected "at risk" situations. At 6 weeks, the DBO was discontinued, and the RMF orthosis and all restrictions were discontinued between 8 and 10 weeks postop.

Passive Motion: Less widely used, these programs involve passive digit flexion with no active contraction of the flexor muscle tendon unit. Wrist position is fixed within a DBO.

Kleinert Program:[11] Introduced in 1977, this program was developed to influence adhesion formation to be elongated and less restrictive. Beginning within 24 hours postop, active blocked and resisted finger extension and passive flexion by elastic traction applied to the nail of the involved and adjacent digits (see **Fig. 1** A, B). Program is advanced at 4 weeks.

Duran protocol:[12] Introduced in 1975, this program was designed for repairs in zone 2 to prevent cross union between the flexor digitorum superficialis (FDS) and FDP. Passive DIP extension with the PIP and MCP flexed glides the FDP suture

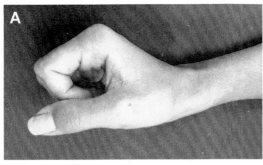
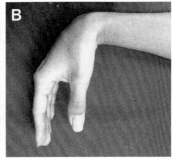

Fig. 9. Synergistic motion[26] is intended to produce a passive proximal glide of the tendon repair site through (*A*) extension of the wrist through a controlled range, resulting in a proximal pull on the tendon with resultant flexion of the digits. (*B*) As the wrist flexes, the fingers extend with the tendon repair site pulled distally.

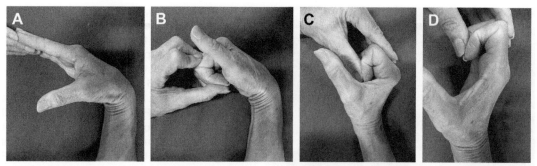

Fig. 10. Modified synergistic motion[27] developed to promote greater proximal pull on the tendon. (A) With the wrist flexed to 60°, passive MCP joint extension and PIP and DIP joints fully extended, the flexor tendon is pulled distally; (B) passive full flexion of the fingers with wrist flexed to 60°; and (C) extension of the wrist to 60° with fingers fully flexed, the tendon is pulled proximally. (D) Gradual extension of the MCP joints to 45° while maintaining flexion of the IP joints.

site away from the FDS suture site. Passive PIP extension with the MCP and DIP flexed glides both suture sites away from the injury site. The program is progressed at 4.5 weeks (see **Fig. 2**).

Washington Regimen:[13] A passive motion protocol that combines the Kleinert and Duran programs (**Fig. 8**).

Synergistic Motion:[26] A passive motion protocol designed to produce a passive proximal glide of the tendon repair site through extension of the wrist through a controlled range, resulting in a proximal pull on the tendon with resultant flexion of the digits. As the wrist flexes, the fingers extend with the tendon repair site pulled distally (**Fig. 9** A,

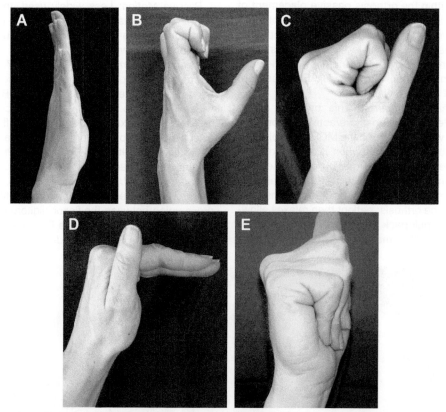

Fig. 11. *Tendon Gliding Exercises described by Hunter and Wehbe*[32,33] based on their study of FDP and FDS tendon gliding and differential gliding in different hand positions: (A) Full finger extension, (B) hook fist, (C) full fist, (D) tabletop position, and (E) straight fist. Hook fist requires maximum differential gliding between the FDS and FDP; full fist requires maximum FDP glide; and straight fist requires maximum FDS glide.

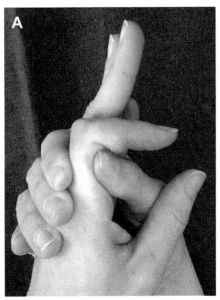
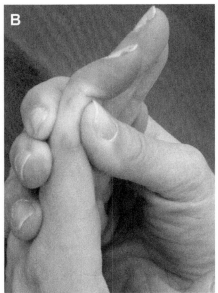

Fig. 12. Isolated joint/blocking exercises. (*A*) Manual or orthotic stabilization of the proximal phalanx with blocking of the MCPJ allows isolated motion of the PIP and DIP joints and promotes differential gliding of the FDP and FDS. (*B*) Manual or orthotic stabilization of the proximal and middle phalanges with blocking of PIP joint motion allows isolated DIP joint motion and promotes FDP glide.

B). *Modification of the synergistic motion approach*[27] was developed to promote greater proximal pull on the tendon by including passive MCP extension following wrist extension (**Fig. 10** A–D).

Initial Immobilization: This protocol allows no active or passive motion for 3 weeks after tendon repair. Used for children or those incapable of complying with the early motion programs, or those with concomitant injuries, which preclude early passive and/or active motion. Cifaldi Collins

and Schwarze[28] developed a protocol for tendons treated with initial immobilization.

CLINICAL REASONING/PROBLEM-SOLVING

Selection of postoperative protocol: In general, it is the surgeon's decision regarding the choice of the postoperative approach, whether passive, active, or active/passive based on the surgical procedure performed and the surgeon's assessment of the capacity of the repair to withstand

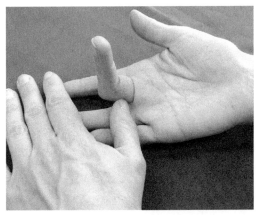

Fig. 13. Isolated FDS glide—Adjacent digits are held in extension with active PIP joint flexion of the involved digit isolating gliding of the FDS.

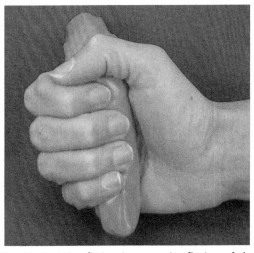

Fig. 14. Resistive fisting is composite flexion of the digits against a resistance such as graded putty.

the forces imparted to the tendon during motion. The knowledgeable therapist, who understands the extent of the injury and the procedures performed, will have valuable input and suggestions regarding the specific protocol chosen and any modifications, the progression of exercises, and feedback regarding the patient's response to therapy. Throughout the rehabilitation process, surgeon–therapist communication and collaboration is critical.

When to Start Motion

The early passive motion programs called for starting motion immediately[29] or within 2 to 3 days[11] after surgery. The more currently used active motion programs typically start within 3 to 5 days after surgery based on studies which examined when following tendon repair the work of flexion (WOF) was the least. WOF refers to the work required of the repaired tendon to actively flex the digit. Tendon loading must be great enough to overcome the WOF but if resistance to motion exceeds the repair strength, rupture or gap formation may occur. Factors that influence the WOF include internal factors such as surface friction and bulk effect of the tendon repair and adhesions and external factors such as edema, joint stiffness, and resistance of antagonist muscles. Zhao and Amadio[30] determined that the WOF was lowest at postoperative day 5 in a canine model with the best combination of tendon tensile strength and low peak resistance force at day 5 and the worst at day 7. Halikis and Manske[31] and colleagues found that a period of delayed mobilization before the institution of active motion protocols is beneficial in decreasing the forces need to flex the digit. Tendons immobilized for 3 days showed the least increase in the WOF compared with those started immediately and at 5 days.

Progression of exercises: The timetables included with the previously described clinical protocols are meant to serve as guidelines and not as rigid prescriptions for when different exercises may be introduced. Rather, clinical judgment and reasoning must be used based on patient's progress or lack of progress. A clinical reasoning approach termed Pyramid of Progressive Force Application has been described by Groth[23] to assist in the progression of exercise after flexor tendon repair. The system consists of a series of 8 exercises in a pyramid format. The base of the pyramid signifies exercises that impart the lowest level of force to the repaired tendon and the pinnacle of the pyramid imparts the maximum loads. Rather than emphasizing the time elapsed since surgery to introduce specific exercises, this model emphasizes a patient's individual tissue response as reflected in tendon excursion. Patients begin exercises at the lowest level and progress upward only as determined necessary to achieve the desired tendon gliding. Progression up the pyramid must be done with care and collaboration between the surgeon and therapist. The levels from least stressful to the most as described by Groth are as follows:

1. Passive protected digital extension
2. Place and hold finger flexion
3. Active composite fist
4. Hook and straight fist[32,33] (**Fig. 11**A–E)
5. Isolated joint motion (blocking (**Fig. 12**A, B; **Fig. 13**).
6. Discontinuation of protective splinting
7. Resistive composite fist—Composite flexion of the digits against a resistance such as graded putty (**Fig. 14**)
8. Resistive hook and straight fist
9. Resisted isolated joint motion

Flexion contractures: Prevention is the best approach through careful orthosis fabrication and positioning of the involved digit. The fit of the DBO must be monitored on an ongoing basis at each therapy visit. If a contracture develops, emphasis can be placed on PIP joint extension

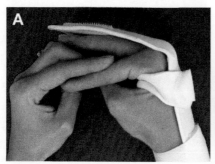
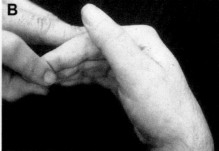

Fig. 15. In the case of a developing PIP joint flexion contracture, emphasis is placed on PIP joint extension performed with (*A*) the MCP joint flexed within a DBO and (*B*) outside of the orthosis.

exercises while the MCP joint is maintained in maximum flexion within the confines of the orthosis (**Fig. 15**).

SUMMARY

Rehabilitation after flexor tendon repairs is a challenging process. The repaired tendon must be simultaneously protected from disruption and moved in a controlled fashion. Although measures are necessary to protect the repaired structures, early controlled motion is required to enhance healing and function. Appropriate intervention at the correct phase of healing is based on an understanding of tendon healing and the factors that influence it. Coordination and communication between the surgeon and therapist is essential. Tendon injuries can profoundly affect hand function and appropriate rehabilitation is essential to preserve function to the fullest extent possible.

CLINICS CARE POINTS

- The goal of therapy after flexor tendon repair is the early restoration of tendon gliding while protecting the repair from rupture.

- The selection of a postoperative protocol after flexor tendon repair whether passive, active or active/passive is based on the surgical procedure performed and the surgeon's assessment of the capacity of the repair to withstand the forces imparted to the tendon during motion.

- Tendon protocols are meant to serve as guidelines and not as rigid timetables. Rather, clinical judgement and reasoning must be used to advance a patient's therapy program and should be based on patient progress or lack of progress.

- Immoderate tendon loading with exercises and use risks tendon rupture and therefore progression of the therapy program after flexor tendon repair must be done with care and collaboration between the surgeon and therapist.

- A not uncommon problem encountered after flexor tendon repair during the rehabilitation process is flexion contracture of the PIP joint of the involved digit. The first and best approach is prevention of contractures by careful orthosis fabrication and positioning of the involved digit. Ongoing monitoring of the fit of the dorsal block orthosis at each therapy visit is essential to prevent loss of appropriate positioning from the reduction in edema and dressings.

ACKNOWLEDGMENTS

None.

REFERENCES

1. Mason JL, Allen HS. The rate of healing tendons: an experimental study of tensile strength. Ann Surg 1941;113(3):424–59.
2. Potenza AD. Clinical evaluation of flexor tendon healing and adhesion formation within artificial digital sheaths: an experimental study. J Bone Joint Surg Am 1963;45A:1217–33.
3. Peacock EE. Biological principles in the healing of long tendons. Surg Clin North Am 1965;45:461–76.
4. Beasley RW. Hand injuries. Philadelphia: WB Saunders; 1981. p. 242–52.
5. Ochiai N, Matsui T, Miyaji N, et al. Vascular anatomy of flexor tendons: Vincular system and blood supply of the profundus tendon in the digital sheath. J Hand Surg Am 1979;4(4):321–30.
6. Manske PR, Bridwell K, Lesker PA. Nutrient pathways to flexor tendons to chickens using tritiated proline. J Hand Surg 1978;3:352–7.
7. Manske PR, Lesker PA, Gelberman RH, et al. Intrinsic restoration of the flexor tendon surface in the nonhuman primate. J Hand Surg Am 1985; 10(5):632–7.
8. Lundborg G, Rank F. Experimental intrinsic healing of flexor tendons based upon synovial fluid nutrition. J Hand Surg 1978;3:21–31.
9. Gelberman RH, Menon J, Gonsalves M, et al. The effects of mobilization on the vascularization of healing tendons in dogs. Clin Orthop 1980;153:283–9.
10. Gelberman RH, Vand Berg JS, Lundberg GH, et al. Flexor tendon healing and restoration of the gliding surface: an ultrastructural study in dogs. J Bone Joint Surg Am 1980;65A:583–95.
11. Lester GD, Kleinert HE, Kutz JE, et al. Primary flexor tendon repair followed by immediate controlled mobilization. J Hand Surg 1977;2A:441–51.
12. Duran RJ, Houser RG. Controlled passive motion following flexor tendon repair in zones 2 and 3. In: American Academy of Orthopedic Surgeons: Symposium on Tendon Surgery in the Hand. St Louis: CV Mosby; 1975.
13. Dovelle S, Heeter PK. The Washington regimen: rehabilitation of the hand following flexor tendon injuries. Phys Ther 1989;69(12):1034–40.
14. Strickland JW, Glogovac SV. Digital function following flexor tendon repair in zone 2: a comparison of immobilization and controlled passive motion techniques. J Hand Surg 1980;5:537–43.
15. Kessler I, Nissim F. Primary repair without immobilization of flexor tendon division within the digital flexor sheath. Acta Orthop Scand 1969;40: 587–601.

16. Strickland JW, Cannon NM. Flexor tendon repair – Indiana Method. Indiana Hand Cent Newsl 1993;1: 1–19.

17. Silfverskiold KL, May EJ. Flexor Tendon repair in zone 2 with a new suture technique and an early mobilization program combining active and passive motion. J Hand Surg 1994;19A:53–60.

18. Evans RB, Thompson DE. Immediate active short arc range of motion following tendon repair. In: Hunter JM, Schneider LH, Mackin EJ, editors. Tendon and nerve surgery in the hand: a third decade. St Louis: CV Mosby; 1997. p. 362–93.

19. Higgins A, Lalonde DH. Flexor tendon repair postoperative rehabilitation: the saint john protocol. Plast Reconstr Surg Glob Open 2016;4:e1134.

20. Tang JB, LaLonde D, Harhaus L, et al. Flexor tendon repair: recent changes and current methods. J Hand Surg 2022;47(1):31–9.

21. Peck FH, Roe AE, Ng CY, et al. The Manchester short splint: a change to splinting practice in the rehabilitation of zone II flexor tendon repairs. Hand Ther 2014;19(2):47–53.

22. Henry SL, Howell JW. Use of a relative motion flexion orthosis for postoperative management of zone I/II flexor digitorum repair: a retrospective case series. J Hand Ther 2019;33(2020):296–304.

23. Groth GN. Pyramid of progressive force exercises to the injured flexor tendon. J Hand Ther 2004;17: 31–42.

24. Strickland JW. Biologic rationale, clinical application and results of early motion following flexor tendon repair. J Hand Ther 1989;2:71–83.

25. Tang JB. Rehabilitation after flexor tendon repair and others: a safe and efficient protocol. J Hand Surg (E) 2021;46(8):813–7.

26. Amadio P. Friction of the gliding surface: Implications for tendon surgery and rehabilitation. J Hand Ther 2005;18(2):112–9.

27. Tanaka T, Amadio P, Zhao C, et al. Flexor digitorum profundus tendon tension during finger manipulation: a study in human cadaver hands. J Hand Ther 2005;18:330–8.

28. Cifaldi-Collins D, Schwarze L. Early Progressive resistance following immobilization of flexor tendon repairs. J Hand Ther 1991;4:111–6.

29. Duran RJ, Coleman CR, Nappi JF, et al. Management of flexor tendon lacerations in zone 2 using controlled passive motion postoperatively. In: Hunter JM, Schneider LH, Mackin EJ, et al, editors. Rehabilitation of the hand: surgery and therapy. third edition. Saint Louis: CV Mosby; 1990. p. 410–3.

30. Zhao C, Amadio PC, Tatsuro T, et al. Short-term assessment of optimal timing for postoperative rehabilitation after flexor digitorum profundus tendon repair in a canine model. J Hand Ther 2005;18:322–8.

31. Halikis MN, Manske PR, Kubota H, et al. Effect of immobilization, immediate mobilization, and delayed mobilization the resistance to digital flexion using a tendon injury model. J Hand Surg 1997;22A:464–72.

32. Wehbe MA, Hunter JM. Flexor tendon gliding in the hand. I. In vivo excursions. J Hand Surg 1985;10:570–5.

33. Wehbe MA, Hunter JM. Flexor tendon gliding in the hand. II. Differential gliding. J Hand Surg 1986;10: 575–9.

Flexor Tendon Reconstruction

Benjamin K. Gundlach, MD[a,b], David S. Zelouf, MD[b,*]

KEYWORDS

- Flexor • Tendon • Reconstruction • Paneva-Holevich

KEY POINTS

- Flexor tendon reconstruction is a challenging problem, with many patients historically achieving poor results.
- Two-stage reconstruction using a silicone rod/device is commonly performed to establish a pseudosheath that can aid in reconstruction.
- With precise technique, a motivated patient, and diligent therapy, functional results can be achieved.

INTRODUCTION

Treatment of flexor tendon injuries has evolved greatly over the last century. Historically it was generally accepted that zone two flexor tendon injuries did poorly after primary repair, and single-stage tendon grafting was the treatment of choice for many surgeons.[1–6] Kleinert's landmark presentation at the 1967 ASSH meeting—where he presented the Louisville experience with primary flexor tendon repair in "no man's land"—ushered in a new era in the field of hand surgery.[7] With modern repair techniques using multi-stranded core sutures and early active motion protocols, outcomes of zone two injuries have greatly improved.[8,9] Despite these advances, a recent meta-analysis by Dy and colleagues[10] showed flexor tendon repair using modern techniques still carries a rupture rate of 4% and rate of reoperation of 6%. In addition, primary flexor tendon repair is not feasible in all patients, including those who present in delayed fashion, with scarring of the tendon sheath, tendon necrosis secondary to pyogenic infection, attritional ruptures, and several other clinical scenarios. It is because of this that flexor tendon reconstruction remains a fundamental—albeit challenging—procedure for the hand surgeon to know and master.

INITIAL EVALUATION AND INDICATIONS

The exact timing around when to consider direct tendon repair versus tendon reconstruction remains unclear. Most would agree that tendon repair within 1 week is ideal, and good to excellent results of primary repair following a delay of 2 to 4 weeks have been published.[11,12] Except in rare circumstances, we believe that delay of 4 weeks or greater leads to musculotendinous retraction and fibrosis, pulley collapse, and digital stiffness, preventing primary repair.

When evaluating a flexor tendon deficient digit, the zone of injury should first be defined. Although flexor tendon reconstruction is performed throughout zones I–V, zone II is the most technically demanding, has the greatest variability in outcomes, and is the zone most focused on in publications regarding reconstruction. Similarly, the mechanism of injury is important to define, as loss of flexor tendon function due to infection or crush injury is more likely to be associated with heavy scar burden compared with a sharp laceration. Lastly, damage to surrounding neurovascular structures should be identified during the initial evaluation. An insensate finger with injury to both digital nerves may be contraindicated for flexor tendon reconstruction owing to poor postoperative outcomes.[13]

[a] Thomas Jefferson University Hospital. Philadelphia, PA, USA; [b] The Philadelphia Hand to Shoulder Center, Thomas Jefferson University Hospital, 834 Chestnut Street, Suite G114, Philadelphia, PA 19107, USA
* Corresponding author.
E-mail address: dszelouf@HANDCENTERS.com

Hand Clin 39 (2023) 193–201
https://doi.org/10.1016/j.hcl.2022.08.020

The management of the finger with an isolated injury to the flexor digitorum profundus (FDP) remains controversial. In the FDP deficient finger, the remaining flexion of the metacarpophalangeal (MCP) joint and proximal interphalangeal (PIP) joint preserves most of the finger's functional motion. Because of this, it has long been held that only in rare circumstances—such as a musician requiring active DIP flexion—should a reconstruction be performed on an isolated FDP injury.[14,15] Instead it is often recommended that the FDP deficient patient who is bothered by a flail distal interphalangeal (DIP) joint undergo a DIP arthrodesis or FDP tenodesis.[16] Good results have been shown with isolated grafting of an FDP through an intact superficialis tendon, and this remains an option in select patients.[17,18]

SINGLE- VERSUS TWO-STAGE RECONSTRUCTION

Once the decision has been made to proceed with flexor tendon reconstruction, the next dilemma becomes whether to perform the single- or two-stage reconstruction. The preoperative condition of the digit, first described by Boyes, remains relevant in clinical decision-making. In his initial series of 138 grafts, Boyes found that the presence of a cicatrix—a dense/deep scar—was associated with the fewest number of patients achieving near-normal digital motion following single-stage tendon grafting.[19] Expanding on his earlier work, Boyes subsequently published his results on 1000 flexor tendon reconstructions, finding that preoperative motion was the most important variable in determining postoperative motion.[20] Therefore, it is recommended that a patient with a stiff digit undergo intensive hand therapy to regain full passive motion before flexor tendon reconstruction.

A set of criteria characterizing the ideal patient for single-stage flexor tendon grafting has been described by Fletcher and McClinton:[14]

1. A committed, motivated patient
2. A finger with full passive motion across all joints
3. Adequate soft-tissue coverage with a soft, mature scar
4. A well-perfused digit with at least one intact digital nerve
5. Minimal to no scarring within the flexor sheath

In patients meeting the above criteria, single-stage reconstruction remains an appropriate, elegant solution, as it typically avoids a secondary reconstructive surgery, and accelerates the patient's recovery/therapy by several months.

SINGLE-STAGE RECONSTRUCTION

The injured finger is approached through either a Brunauer or midaxial incision, allowing access to the injured flexor tendons which are then excised. It is important to never sacrifice or excise a functioning FDS tendon. A small stump of FDP tendon is left remaining at the distal phalanx to reinforce the distal tenorrhaphy. The pulley system must not be injured or compromised throughout the surgical procedure, as this risks bowstringing, adhesion formation, and potential failure of the single-stage reconstruction.

A tendon graft is harvested, temporarily sewn to a pediatric feeding tube, and then passed through the pulley system using the feeding tube as a shuttle. The graft is first fixed distally to the FDP stump and distal phalanx using the surgeon's preferred technique. Next, using the surgeon's preferred tendon weave technique, the proximal extent of the graft is woven into the proximal stump of the FDP tendon, and appropriate tension is set to establish a natural digital cascade and tenodesis. Two or three additional tendon weaves are performed to secure the proximal tenorrhaphy site.

Because the distal tenorrhaphy site is often the weakest link in either a single or two-stage reconstruction, our preference is to complete this step first, and the proximal tenorrhaphy second. This allows for the distal fixation to be performed with the finger extended, providing full access to the distal phalanx and FDP stump. In addition, the tension on the graft can be adjusted easier as the weave can be released and reset. Based on our experience, an over- or under-tensioned graft is more difficult to adjust at the distal site.

Multiple techniques have been described for distal fixation of the tendon to phalanx. Classically, running locked grasping sutures are placed along the tendon, holes drilled through the distal phalanx, the sutures then placed through the holes in a volar to dorsal direction, and tied directly over the fingernail or a dorsal button. With this technique it is important to avoid violating the germinal matrix with the drill or sutures, instead exiting within the sterile matrix. More recently, miniature suture anchors have gained popularity as an all-internal fixation option, with the main benefit of avoiding the dorsal button/knots while also providing strong fixation with less tendon gap formation.[21–23]

Because the small, ring, and middle finger share a common profundus muscle belly, it is important to not over-tension the graft and causes quadrigia. In addition, if performing the proximal tenorrhaphy in the palm, it is important to maximally extend the digit before finalizing the tenorrhaphy to ensure the bulky tendon weave will not impinge on the flexor sheath. It may be necessary to divide the A1 pulley if this is encountered.

A unique example of single-stage reconstruction is the flexor pollicis longus (FPL) (**Fig. 1**). Because the thumb has a much simpler pulley system and requires less total active motion (TAM) than the fingers, single-stage reconstruction of the FPL often produces good to excellent functional results.[20,24] This can either be accomplished with a tendon bridge graft (see **Fig. 1**B), or a ring FDS tendon transfer. The thumb distal phalanx is more proximal in the hand when compared with the middle phalanx of the ring finger; therefore, the FPL tendon is also shorter in length compared with the FDS tendon. When transferring an FDS, this allows the surgeon to release the FDS proximal to its terminal insertion—avoiding unnecessary injury to the vinculum—while maintaining more than enough length to reach the thumb distal phalanx.[25,26]

For flexor tendon disruption within zones III—V, single-stage bridge grafting of the tendon defect can be accomplished with good results.[27–29]

In either single or two-stage reconstruction, we believe early active motion should begin soon after the terminal surgery to limit the re-formation of joint contractures and the development of tendon adhesions. If the proximal or distal tenorrhaphy site was performed under tenuous conditions, or there are concerns for repair site gapping, active motion should be delayed to prevent graft rupture. Many different protocols have been described in the acute flexor tendon population that can be readily adapted to the reconstructed population.

GRAFT CHOICE

With rare exception, flexor tendon reconstruction is performed with autograft tissue. Described graft sources are numerous, and often are determined by what donor tendons are available. When the proximal tendon-tendon interface is within the palm—such as with zone two reconstructions—the palmaris longus (PL) is frequently used as it is often available within the same operative field, has acceptable length, and adequate strength.[24] Absence of the PL is estimated to occur in 10% to 15% of individuals, and with considerable geographic variance in the rate of agenesis.[30,31] With proximal reconstruction at the level of the wrist, or when the PL is absent, the plantaris tendon is commonly used, although there is also wide variability in the described rate of agenesis and location of insertion of the plantaris.[24,32,33]

PL and plantaris are both considered extrasynovial tendons, because in their native state they are not contained within a tenosynovial sheath and do not contain a vascularized epitenon. Intrasynovial tendons, such as flexor tendons, do contain a vascularized epitenon.[34] Other extrasynovial tendons that have been used to reconstruct flexor tendons include toe extensors, extensor indicis proprius, and semitendinosus, among others.[34,35] Flexor tendon reconstruction with extrasynovial grafting, even when performed by experienced surgeons, is frequently complicated by adhesions and the need to perform secondary tenolysis.[36] Owing to this, the use of intrasynovial graft has been investigated, finding in a canine animal model that intrasynovial toe-flexor grafts formed fewer adhesions and were associated with less tendon necrosis following grafting.[37,38] Clinically, the use of toe-flexors has been shown to be feasible, with little donor-site morbidity and a low rate of adhesion formation; however, no direct clinical comparisons have been made between extrasynovial and intrasynovial grafts (**Fig. 2**).[39,40]

A variant of intrasynovial tendon grafting is using the proximal stump of the injured FDS tendon during a two-stage reconstruction, as initially described by Paneva-Holvich (**Figs. 3** and **4**). With this technique, during the first stage of tendon reconstruction a silicone rod is placed along the flexor sheath, and the distal ends of both the FDS and FDP are sutured together using the surgeon's preferred tenorrhaphy technique (see

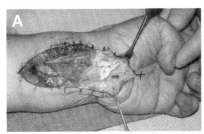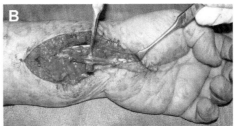

Fig. 1. (*A*) An attritional rupture of the flexor pollicis longus (FPL) following hardware removal of the volar distal radius. Arrows indicate proximal and distal FPL. (*B*) The damaged segment of FPL is reconstructed using palmaris longus bridge graft.

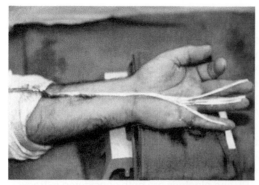

Fig. 2. A three-tailed graft harvested from the toe flexor digitorum longus used to reconstruct a chronic small, ring, and middle finger flexor tendon injury.

Fig. 3). At the second stage, the affected FDS is then released at the musculotendinous junction proximally, and then retrieved in the wrist or palm (see **Fig. 4**A). The previous FDS-FDP tenorrhaphy—now united—allows the FDS tendon to serve as an intrasynovial tendon graft/extension off the FDP. The FDS is sutured to the silicone rod, pulled through the healed flexor sheath, and fixed to the distal phalanx (see **Fig. 4**B) using either a dorsal button, a suture anchor within the distal phalanx, or a combination of techniques.[41] The

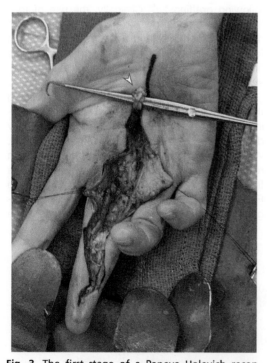

Fig. 3. The first stage of a Paneva–Holevich reconstruction. The FDP-FDS tenorrhaphy can be seen wrapping around the silver retractor. A silicone rod was subsequently placed, and pulleys reconstructed.

primary difficulty with this operation is setting appropriate tension, as the digital cascade cannot be assessed fully until after the graft has been sutured and fixed into position.

Use of allograft tendon to reconstruct a flexor tendon was first described in 1967 by Peacock and Madden. They presented results of 10 patients who underwent fresh allograft flexor tendon composite grafting which included the tendon along with the pulley system, with good results.[42] Concerns regarding disease transmission and tissue processing, however, have dampened clinical adoption of this technique. More recently, animal research has expanded on this to improve allograft tendon strength, gliding, and reduce adhesions; however, concerns still remain about allograft tendon's ability to form the solid tendon-to-bone healing required at the distal junction of a flexor tendon reconstruction.[43–48] Limited clinical data are available on the use of allograft tendon for flexor tendon reconstruction. Xie and Tang[49] published on 22 patients undergoing 30 allograft reconstructions with good results. Their study, however, did not include objective data on long-term outcomes. Wang and colleagues[50] published on ten patients who received 26 allograft tendon reconstructions following severe hand trauma with an average of 50 months follow-up. They reported a mean TAM of 126°, and only one case of tendon adhesion. More recently the use of composite allografts composed of either bone-tendon, or bone-tendon-flexor sheath has been investigated as a potential off-the-shelf product for flexor tendon reconstruction. At this time there are no clinical data available yet.[51,52]

TWO-STAGE RECONSTRUCTION

If the conditions allowing for single-stage tendon grafting are not met, then two-stage flexor tendon reconstruction is required. The technique of two-stage reconstruction remains largely unchanged from the one described by Hunter and Salisbury.[53] The first stage involves excision of all scarred and necrotic tendon and sheath within the zone of injury, release of any contracted joints, repair or reconstruction of injured digital nerves, pulley reconstruction as necessary, and placement of a silicone implant (**Fig. 5**). This often requires an extensile exposure along the entire digit and palm, and another incision proximal to the carpal tunnel to retrieve the silicone rod. To facilitate gliding of the silicone rod, it should be placed through the carpal tunnel and into the distal forearm, even when reconstructing a zone I–III defect, as an implant ending within the palm may kink or buckle and prevent gliding. A 1 cm stump of FDP

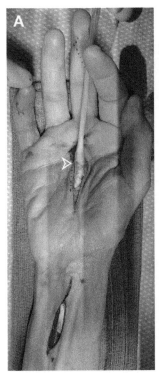
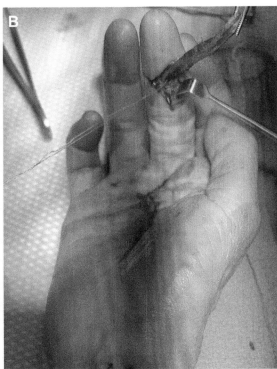

Fig. 4. (*A*) The second stage Paneva–Holevich reconstruction. The FDS tendon was released proximally, and the entire tendon unit retrieved (*arrow*). The tenorrhaphy site is well healed. (*B*) The tendon is then pulled through the digit and fixed to the distal phalanx using suture anchors.

is left attached to the distal phalanx, and the distal end of the silicone implant is sewn to the tendon stump and adjacent volar plate with 3 to 0 nonabsorbable suture. The silicone rod is left unattached proximally, as the goal of the rod is to enhance sheath formation, rather than to serve as an active prosthesis.

Postoperatively the patient is started in supervised hand therapy to begin passive motion exercises, including learning to trap the affected finger with the adjacent digits and flex it into the palm. We recommend the second stage be delayed until tissue equilibrium has been reached, meaning there is full passive motion with a soft, mature scar. We generally find this does not occur sooner than 8 weeks from the first stage.

At the second stage of reconstruction, a more limited exposure is performed. Re-exposing or violating the pulley system and pseudosheath is to be avoided. The site of the planned proximal tenorrhaphy is approached, the pseudosheath incised, and the silicone implant retrieved at this level. A limited approach is then used to expose the distal phalanx and FDP tendon stump. A tendon graft is then sewn to the rod proximally, and by pulling traction on the distal aspect of the

rod, the tendon graft is pulled through the pseudosheath and pulley system and introduced into the distal incision. Hemostats should then be placed proximally and distally to control the silicone-tendon unit and prevent inadvertent pull-out of the construct. With the graft in place distal tenorrhaphy is performed first, followed by the proximal tenorrhaphy, per surgeon preference as previously discussed.

Hunter and his team discussed their initial clinical results in 69 fingers (Boyes grades 2, 3, and 5) undergoing two-stage reconstruction, with 25% of patients achieving full passive motion, and 57% of patients achieving active flexion to within 1.3 cm or less pulp-to-crease.[53] These results were then followed with their 10-year experience with two-stage reconstruction on 136 patients. On average, patients improved from a TAM before surgery of 102° to 176° following two reconstructions. Of note, 12.4% of fingers required reoperation for tenolysis, and 14.1% for repair of a ruptured tendon graft.[54] Similar results have been found by other authors, with an average of only 50% of patients achieving a good or excellent result, and with infection, stiffness requiring tenolysis, and rupture as common complications.[55,56]

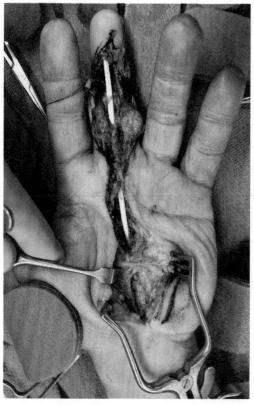

Fig. 5. A middle finger that underwent previous replantation, with subsequent failure of the flexor tendon repair with dense adhesions. The flexor tendons were excised, A2 and A4 pulley maintained, and a silicone rod placed.

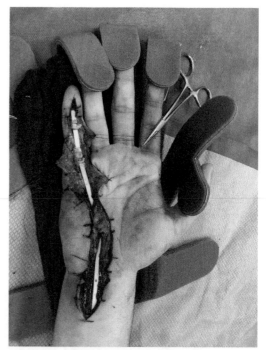

Fig. 6. A small finger with complete deficiency of the pulley system. A silicone rod was placed, and the A2 and A4 pulleys reconstructed using remnant FDS tendon in a wrap-around technique.

SILICONE ROD MECHANISM OF ACTION

The use of flexible silicone implants was first described by Carroll and Bassett in 1963 as a method to induce the formation of a pseudosheath in a digit that was otherwise traumatized and contraindicated for primary grafting.[57] This work was further expanded on by Hunter in 1965 using silicone rods reinforced with dacron fiber, showing that the use of reinforced silicone rods creates an environment more accepting of a tendon graft, with less scarring and improved gliding characteristics.[58] The pseudosheath that forms following implantation of a silicone implant is different than a true mesothelial lined tenosynovial sheath. Instead, the pseudosheath is rich in fibroblast activity, a capillary network that peaks in vascularity around 4 to 6 weeks, and a rudimentary secretory ability of a synovial-like fluid.[59–61] Although a pseudosheath beings to form within 7 to 14 days following silicone rod placement, because of the strong fibroblastic and angiogenic activity during the first 6 weeks it is recommend to avoid tendon grafting during this time to decrease the risk of fibrosis/adhesions.[60]

PULLEY MANAGEMENT

In the setting of complete rupture or incompetence of the pulley system, reconstruction should be performed to prevent bowstringing and improve the mechanical action of the flexor tendon reconstruction. Several reconstructive methods have been described using a variety of graft materials and various constructs. Kleinert and Bennet described a technique using a free tendon graft, creating a weave across the "ever-present" rims of pulley that often remain even following severe trauma or infection.[62] Lister described using a slip of extensor retinaculum wrapped circumferentially around the phalanx.[63] Karev described a technique using a belt-loop using a slip of volar plate.[64] Several techniques have described using a tendon graft and creating a loop/s around the phalax.[65] Comparing many of these techniques together, Widstrom and colleagues[65,66] found that the Karev technique of volar plate "belt-loops" was the most mechanically effective, whereas a "loop and one-half" reconstruction was the strongest. In a separate study, Lister's technique of using an intrasynovial graft from the extensor retinaculum had the lowest resistance of tendon gliding.[67] In addition, the use of allograft pulley system has been shown clinically with good results.[68] Alternatively, the ruptured flexor tendon that is excised may be used with a variety of the above techniques to reconstruct the pulleys, avoiding the need to harvest additional autograft material.

The effect that that partial loss of the pulley system has on the development of bowstringing and loss of motion remains unclear. In the setting of primary repair, a limited pulley release—commonly referred to as "venting"—is performed to allow for end-to-end repair. Under this circumstance it has been shown that complete release of either the A2 or A4 pulley, in combination with their immediately adjacent cruciate pulley, has little effect on the development of clinical bowstringing.[69–72] Although not tested in the setting of flexor tendon reconstruction, these results call into question the necessity of reconstructing an A2 or A4 pulley in isolation if the much of the pulley system remains intact. In the setting of complete, or near-complete pulley loss, we still recommend reconstruction of the A2 and A4 pulleys (**Fig. 6**).

SUMMARY

Despite nearly a century passing since the field's pioneers first described their reconstructive efforts, flexor tendon reconstruction remains an unyielding technical and rehabilitative challenge for the modern hand surgeon and therapist. Using many of the same principles developed by Drs Bunnell, Boyes, Pulvertaft, Hunter, Schneider, and others, this difficult patient population can often achieve functional results. Prospective studies are still needed to clarify lingering questions such as intrasynovial versus extrasynovial tendon grafting. In addition, basic science investigations into the use of tendon modifiers to decrease adhesion formation, or the processing and use of allograft tendon, are potential areas to improve the clinical care of this patient population.

CLINICS CARE POINTS

- Preoperative motion predicts postoperative motion. Although it is tempting for both surgeon and patient to proceed swiftly through each stage of reconstruction, it is critically important that full passive motion be achieved prior to each stage of surgery.

- Wide Awake Local Anesthesia No Tourniquet (WALANT) can allow intraoperative testing of the flexor tendon repair/reconstruction site, allowing the surgeon to observe for tenorrhaphy gapping, or catching/buckling within the flexor sheath, and address these issues in real time.

- Tendon adhesion is not uncommon, especially following two-stage flexor tendon reconstructions. A patient who has full passive motion but poor active motion, and who has plateaued with therapy, may be indicated for tenolysis.

DISCLOSURE

None.

REFERENCES

1. Boyes JH. Why Tendon Repair? J Bone Joint Surg Am 1959;41(4):577–9.
2. Posch J. Primary Tenorrhaphies and Tendon Grafting Procedures in Hand Injuries. AMA Arch Surg 1956;73(4):609–24.
3. Siler VE. Primary Tenorrhaphy of the Flexor Tendons in the Hand. J Bone Joint Surg Am 1950;32(1):218–25.
4. Mason ML. Primary Tendon Repair. J Bone Joint Surg Am 1959;41(4):575–7.
5. Kelly APJ. Primary Tendon Repairs: A Study of 789 Consecutive Tendon Severances. J Bone Joint Surg Am 1959;41(4):581–664.
6. Bunnell S. Repair of Tendons in the Fingers and Descriptions of Two New Instruments. Surg Gynecol Obstet 1918;26:103–10.
7. Kleinert HE, Kutz JE, Ashbell TS, et al. Primary Repair of Lacerated Flexor Tendons in "No Man's Land. J Bone Joint Surg Am 1967;49(3):577.
8. Tang JB. Outcomes and Evaluation of Flexor Tendon Repair. Hand Clin 2013;29(2):251–9.
9. Starnes T, Saunders RJ, Means KR. Clinical Outcomes of Zone II Flexor Tendon Repair Depending on Mechanism of Injury. J Hand Surg 2012;37(12):2532–40.
10. Dy CJ, Hernandez-Soria A, Ma Y, et al. Complications After Flexor Tendon Repair: A Systematic Review and Meta-Analysis. J Hand Surg Am 2012;37(3):543–51.e1.
11. Tang J. Indications, Methods, Postoperative Motion and Outcome Evaluation of Primary Flexor Tendon Repairs in Zone 2. J Hand Surg Eur 2007;32(2):118–29.
12. Munz G, Poggetti A, Cenci L, et al. Up to five-week delay in primary repair of Zone 2 flexor tendon injuries: outcomes and complications. J Hand Surg Eur 2021;46(8):818–24.

13. Schneider LH. Staged flexor tendon reconstruction using the method of Hunter. Clin Orthop Relat Res 1982;171:164–71.

14. Fletcher DR, McClinton MA. Single-Stage Flexor Tendon Grafting: Refining the Steps. J Hand Surg Am 2015;40(7):1452–60.

15. Holm CL, Embick RP. Anatomical considerations in the primary treatment of tendon injuries of the hand. J Bone Joint Surg Am 1959;41-A(4):599–608.

16. Kahn S. A dynamic tenodesis of the distal interphalangeal joint, for use after severance of the profundus alone. Plast Reconstr Surg 1973;51(5):536–40.

17. McClinton MA, Curtis RM, Wilgis EFS. One hundred tendon grafts for isolated flexor digitorum profundus injuries. J Hand Surg Am 1982;7(3):224–9.

18. Pulvertaft RG. The Treatment of Profundus Division by Free Tendon Graft. J Bone Joint Surg Am 1960; 42(8):1363–80.

19. Boyes JH. Flexor Tendon Grafts in the Fingers and Thumb: An Evaluation of End Results. J Bone Joint Surg Am 1950;32(3):489–531.

20. Boyes JH, Stark HH. Flexor-Tendon Grafts in the Fingers and Thumb: A Study of Factors Influencing Results in 1000 Cases. J Bone Joint Surg Am 1971; 53(7):1332–42.

21. Matsuzaki H, Zaegel MA, Gelberman RH, et al. Effect of Suture Material and Bone Quality on the Mechanical Properties of Zone I Flexor Tendon–Bone Reattachment With Bone Anchors. J Hand Surg Am 2008;33(5):709–17.

22. Brustein M, Pellegrini J, Choueka J, et al. Bone suture anchors versus the pullout button for repair of distal profundus tendon injuries: A comparison of strength in human cadaveric hands. J Hand Surg Am 2001;26(3):489–96.

23. Chu JY, Chen T, Awad HA, et al. Comparison of All-Inside Suture Technique with Traditional Pull-out Suture and Suture Anchor Repair Techniques for Flexor Digitorum Profundus Attachment to Bone. J Hand Surg Am 2013;38(6):1084–90.

24. Pulvertaft RG. Tendon grafts for flexor tendon injuries in the fingers and thumb; a study of technique and results. J Bone Joint Surg Br 1956;38-B(1): 175–94.

25. Posner MA. Flexor superficialis tendon transfers to the thumb–an alternative to the free tendon graft for treatment of chronic injuries within the digital sheath. J Hand Surg Am 1983;8(6):876–81.

26. Schneider LH, Wiltshire D. Restoration of flexor pollicis longus function by flexor digitorum superficialis transfer. J Hand Surg Am 1983;8(1):98–101.

27. Stark HH, Anderson DR, Zemel NP, et al. Bridge flexor tendon grafts. Clin Orthop Relat Res 1989;(242):51–9.

28. Kuroda T, Moriya K, Tsubokawa N, et al. Comparison of bridge graft and end-to-side transfer for treatment of closed rupture of the flexor tendons in the little finger. J Hand Surg Eur 2022;47(5):520–6.

29. Kim YJ, Baek JH, Park JS, et al. Interposition Tendon Graft and Tension in the Repair of Closed Rupture of the Flexor Digitorum Profundus in Zone III or IV. Ann Plast Surg 2018;80(3):238–41.

30. Reimann AF, Daseler EH, Anson BJ, et al. The palmaris longus muscle and tendon. A study of 1600 extremities. Anatomical Rec 1944;89(4):495–505.

31. Ioannis D, Anastasios K, Konstantinos N, et al. Palmaris Longus Muscle's Prevalence in Different Nations and Interesting Anatomical Variations: Review of the Literature. J Clin Med Res 2015;7(11):825–30.

32. Meyer P, Pesquer L, Boudahmane S, et al. Evaluation of the plantaris tendon: cadaver anatomy study with ultrasonographic and clinical correlation with tennis leg injury in 759 calves. Skeletal Radiol 2022;51(9):1797–806.

33. Spang C, Alfredson H, Docking SI, et al. The plantaris tendon. Bone Joint J 2016;98-B(10):1312–9.

34. Wong R, Alam N, McGrouther AD, et al. Tendon grafts: their natural history, biology and future development. J Hand Surg Eur 2015;40(7):669–81.

35. Low N, Fahy ET, Frisken J, et al. An alternate graft for staged flexor tendon reconstruction. Hand (N Y). 2015;10(1):152–4.

36. LaSalle WB, Strickland JW. An evaluation of the two-stage flexor tendon reconstruction technique. J Hand Surg 1983;8(3):263–7.

37. Abrahamsson SO, Gelberman RH, Lohmander SL. Variations in cellular proliferation and matrix synthesis in intrasynovial and extrasynovial tendons: An in vitro study in dogs. J Hand Surg Am 1994;19(2): 259–65.

38. Ark JW, Gelberman RH, Abrahamsson SO, et al. Cellular survival and proliferation in autogenous flexor tendon grafts. J Hand Surg Am 1994;19(2): 249–58.

39. Sasaki J, Itsubo T, Nakamura K, et al. Intrasynovial Tendon Graft for Chronic Flexor Tendon Laceration of the Finger: A Case Report. Open Orthop J 2013;7:282–5.

40. Leversedge FJ, Zelouf D, Williams C, et al. Flexor tendon grafting to the hand: An assessment of the intrasynovial donor tendon—A preliminary single-cohort study. J Hand Surg Am 2000;25(4):721–30.

41. Paneva-Holevich E. Two-Stage Tenoplasty in Injury of the Flexor Tendons of the Hand. J Bone Joint Surg Am 1969;51(1):21–32.

42. Peacock EE, Madden JW. Human composite flexor tendon allografts. Ann Surg 1967;166(4):624–9.

43. Zhao C, Sun YL, Amadio PC, et al. Surface Treatment of Flexor Tendon Autografts with Carbodiimide-Derivatized Hyaluronic Acid. J Bone Joint Surg Am 2006;88(10):2181–91.

44. Zhang T, Lu CC, Reisdorf RL, et al. Revitalized and synovialized allograft for intrasynovial flexor tendon

reconstruction in an in vivo canine model. J Orthop Res 2018;36(8):2218–27.

45. Ikeda J, Zhao C, Sun YL, et al. Carbodiimide-Derivatized Hyaluronic Acid Surface Modification of Lyophilized Flexor Tendon. J Bone Joint Surg Am 2010;92(2):388–95.

46. Chang J. Studies in Flexor Tendon Reconstruction: Biomolecular Modulation of Tendon Repair and Tissue Engineering. J Hand Surg Am 2012;37(3): 552–61.

47. Potenza AD, Melone C. Evaluation of freeze-dried flexor tendon grafts in the dog. J Hand Surg Am 1978;3(2):157–62.

48. Wei Z, Reisdorf RL, Thoreson AR, et al. Comparison of Autograft and Allograft with Surface Modification for Flexor Tendon Reconstruction. J Bone Joint Surg Am 2018;100(7):e42.

49. Xie RG, Tang JB. Allograft Tendon for Second-Stage Tendon Reconstruction. Hand Clin 2012;28(4): 503–9.

50. Wang GH, Mao T, Xing SG, et al. Functional reconstruction of severe hand injuries using allogeneic tendons: a retrospective study. J Int Med Res 2020;48(10). 0300060520955032.

51. Fox PM, Farnebo S, Lindsey D, et al. Decellularized Human Tendon–Bone Grafts for Composite Flexor Tendon Reconstruction: A Cadaveric Model of Initial Mechanical Properties. J Hand Surg Am 2013; 38(12):2323–8.

52. DeGeorge BRJ, Rodeheaver GT, Drake DB. The Biophysical Characteristics of Human Composite Flexor Tendon Allograft for Upper Extremity Reconstruction. Ann Plast Surg 2014;72(6):S184–90.

53. Hunter JM, Salisbury RE. Flexor-Tendon Reconstruction in Severely Damaged Hands: A Two-Stage Procedure Using a Silicone-Dacron Reinforced Gliding Prosthesis Prior to Tendon Grafting. J Bone Joint Surg Am 1971;53(5):829–58.

54. Wehbé MA, Mawr B, Hunter JM, et al. Two-stage flexor-tendon reconstruction. Ten-year experience. J Bone Joint Surg Am 1986;68(5):752–63.

55. Amadio PC, Wood MB, Cooney WP, et al. Staged flexor tendon reconstruction in the fingers and hand. J Hand Surg 1988;13(4):559–62.

56. Coyle MP, Leddy TP, Leddy JP. Staged flexor tendon reconstruction fingertip to palm. J Hand Surg 2002; 27(4):581–5.

57. Bassett CA, Carroll RE. Formation of a tendon sheath by silicone-rod implants. J Bone Joint Surg Am 1963;45(4):884–5.

58. Hunter JM. Artificial Tendons-Their Early Development and Application. In Proceedings of the American Society for Surgery of the Hand. J Bone Joint Surg Am 1965;47(3):631–2.

59. Farkas LG, McCain WG, Sweeney P, et al. An experimental study of the changes following silastic rod preparation of a new tendon sheath and subsequent tendon grafting. J Bone Joint Surg Am 1973;55(6): 1149–58.

60. Rayner CRW. The origin and nature of pseudosynovium appearing around implanted silastic rods an experimental study. The Hand 1976;8(2):101–9.

61. Hunter JM, Subin D, Minkow F, et al. Sheath formation in response to limited active gliding implants (animals). J Biomed Mater Res 1974;8(3):163–73.

62. Klinert HE, Bennett JB. Digital pulley reconstruction employing the always present rim of the previous pulley. J Hand Surg Am 1978;3(3):297–8.

63. Lister GD. Reconstruction of pulleys employing extensor retinaculum. J Hand Surg Am 1979;4(5): 461–4.

64. Karev A. The "belt loop" technique for the reconstruction of pulleys in the first stage of flexor tendon grafting. J Hand Surg Am 1984;9(6):923–4.

65. Widstrom CJ, Johnson G, Doyle JR, et al. A mechanical study of six digital pulley reconstruction techniques: Part I. Mechanical effectiveness. J Hand Surg Am 1989;14(5):821–5.

66. Widstrom CJ, Doyle JR, Johnson G, et al. A mechanical study of six digital pulley reconstruction techniques: Part II. Strength of individual reconstructions. J Hand Surg Am 1989;14(5):826–9.

67. Nishida J, Amadio PC, Bettinger PC, et al. Flexor tendon-pulley interaction after pulley reconstruction: a biomechanical study in a human model in vitro. J Hand Surg Am 1998;23(4):665–72.

68. Martinez RA, Liston J, Archual AJ, et al. Digital Pulley Reconstruction Using Pulley Allografts: A Comparison With Traditional Tendon-Based Techniques. Ann Plast Surg 2019;82(6S):S386–8.

69. Tang JB. Release of the A4 pulley to facilitate zone II flexor tendon repair. J Hand Surg Am 2014;39(11): 2300–7.

70. Moriya K, Yoshizu T, Tsubokawa N, et al. Outcomes of release of the entire A4 pulley after flexor tendon repairs in zone 2A followed by early active mobilization. J Hand Surg Eur 2016;41(4):400–5.

71. Moriya K, Yoshizu T, Tsubokawa N, et al. Clinical results of releasing the entire A2 pulley after flexor tendon repair in zone 2C. J Hand Surg Eur 2016; 41(8):822–8.

72. Tang JB. How to vent the pulley properly without tendon bowstringing in zone 2 repair. Chirurgie de la Main 2015;34(6):395–6.

Tenolysis and Salvage Procedures

David Cholok, MD[a],*, Jordan Burgess, BA[a], Paige M. Fox, MD, PhD[a,b], James Chang, MD[a,b]

KEYWORDS

- Two-staged flexor tendon reconstruction • Flexor tenolysis • Tendon rupture • Adhesion formation
- Joint contracture

KEY POINTS

- Complications in primary flexor tendon repair are common and include tendon rupture, adhesion formation, and joint contracture.
- Rupture of a repaired tendon should be treated by early operative exploration, debridement, and revision with a four-core strand suture and nonbraided epitendinous suture.
- Adhesion formation may be mitigated with the use of epitendinous and core sutures, and early postoperative mobilization.
- Flexor tenolysis should be considered if the range of motion has plateaued and passive motion exceeds active motion.
- Staged reconstruction is recommended when injury results in excessive scaring, joint contracture, or an incompetent pully apparatus.

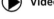 Video content accompanies this article at http://www.hand.theclinics.com.

INTRODUCTION

Tendon lacerations remain a significant public health burden, occurring at an estimated incidence of 33.2 persons per 100,000 per year, resulting in significant morbidity and time off work.[1] Generally, more than 75% of flexor digitorum profundus (FDP) tendon laceration repairs within zones I and II yield functionally favorable results in both adults and children.[2–4] Yet, functionally reliable repair of flexor tendon injuries remains difficult, despite improvements in our understanding of the biomechanics and physiology of tendon healing[5]; indeed, up to 6% to 17% of patients require reoperation, including, most commonly, flexor tenolysis to provide an optimized result.[2,6,7] Challenges in primary repairs are precipitated by concurrent and, unfortunately, competing forces required to reestablish not only tendon continuity but also gliding with minimal friction within the surrounding fibro-osseous canal of the tendon, a balance which is difficult to achieve.[8,9]

Success of repair, and by extension, the risk that a complication may arise, is dependent on patient-specific and technical factors; these can be further subdivided into pre-operative, intraoperative, and postoperative factors. Patient-specific, preoperative risks for inferior outcomes include preexisting comorbid conditions which may affect wound healing, including diabetes mellitus. Circumstances and mechanism of injury should also be taken into consideration by the surgeon; gross contamination of the injury site can predispose to infection and wound breakdown. Concurrent

a Division of Plastic and Reconstructive Surgery, Stanford University Medical Center, 770 Welch Road, Suite 400, Palo Alto, CA 94304, USA; b Division of Plastic and Reconstructive Surgery, Chase Hand and Upper Limb Center, Stanford University Medical Center, 770 Welch Road, Suite 400, Palo Alto, CA 94304, USA
* Corresponding author.
E-mail address: Dcholok@stanford.edu

Hand Clin 39 (2023) 203–214
https://doi.org/10.1016/j.hcl.2022.08.021

fracture and soft-tissue loss may also influence the success of repair via technical considerations and timing of postoperative rehabilitation initiation.

Intraoperative factors, including data-driven technical refinements, have also improved postoperative complications. The use of a minimum of 4 core strand sutures has decreased rates of rupture, especially in the setting of early active range of motion protocols for rehabilitation.[10] In addition, the use of an epitendinous suture is suspected to confer improved tendon gliding and 25% of repair strength.[11–13] More recently, selective venting of pulleys and the preference to forego repair of a ruptured flexor digitorum superficialis (FDS) tendon in Zone II have been demonstrated to limit the obstruction of tendon gliding within the fibro-osseous tunnel at the theoretic risk of tendon bowstringing and diminished strength of the repair, respectively.[14–16]

Postoperative rehabilitation and dedicated participation of the patient are equally essential to the success of flexor tendon repair. Despite the myriad of rehabilitation protocols in existence, no single regimen has been shown to be superior to another; however, there is consensus that prolonged immobilization and poor compliance with early range of motion rehabilitation protocols yield inferior functional results.[17] Early motion protocols confer superior outcomes via minimizing extrinsic scarring and adhesion formation, increasing ultimate tensile load over time, and improving vascular perfusion and synovial fluid distribution to the tendon.[18–21] There has been much debate and change in trends between the prioritization of active versus passive range of motion in the early postoperative period. With stronger, sleeker repairs, early active motion regimens have become increasingly standard and effective; a recent systematic review demonstrated improved greater total active motion when compared with passive range of motion protocols at the conclusion of rehabilitation, although at the cost of increased tendon rupture if repaired with only 2-core strands.[10]

Despite the mitigation of potential risk factors, poor outcomes can and will occur. It is incumbent on the surgeon to be able to assess for suboptimal results and to be able to perform revision procedures to restore the best functional outcome possible.

Early Complications

Infection

Infection following surgical flexor tendon repair is rare and can be related to the degree of contamination conferred by the precipitating trauma, as well as inadequate irrigation and debridement.[22] Following standard reconstructive principles, any repair should only be performed in a clean wound. Scenarios in which surgeons should be particularly attuned to an increased risk of infection include replantation, injuries in the maritime or agricultural settings, bite wounds, and delayed repair of an open wound. Inadequate debridement, such as in the setting of crush injuries or open fracture, may also predispose to infection. It should be noted that routine peri-operative IV antibiotic administration does not mitigate the risk of perioperative infection; it bears repeating that only adequate debridement and irrigation are prerequisite to ensure minimal risk of subsequent infection.[23]

Fortunately, the incidence of infection following tendon repair is rare, and occurs at a rate of approximately 2%.[23] Treatment of infectious complications should follow standard principles including early initiation of antibiotics and operative drainage of any deep-space abscess or fluid collection. Prompt the recognition of infection and avoidance of treatment delay will improve time to infection resolution.[24] Nonviable tissue, when present, should be adequately debrided. To that end, initial laceration and any planned incisions should take into consideration in designing skin flaps without narrow tips, as careless skin incisions may result in devascularized tissue. Preexisting lacerations can often be incorporated into midlateral, or Brunauer incisions to minimize the risk of flexion contracture. The tendon repair itself should be carefully examined for the need to reinforce the repair or to debride the tendon and proceed to later staged tendon reconstruction. Gross soft tissue loss can be replaced with tissue transfer via local, regional, or free-tissue transfer, including venous flaps.

Flexor tendon rupture

Tendons are hypocellular and heal by both intrinsic and extrinsic cellular pathways, following an established paradigm of 3 overlapping stages of inflammation, proliferation, and remodeling.[25,26] Concordant with these phases, primary repair of lacerated tendons is most susceptible to rupture at days 6 to 18 postoperatively, as the initial strength of the suture degrades and the transition from the proliferative to the remodeling phase has yet to yield an optimal orientation of collagen fibers.[27] Though rare, ruptures occurring years after repair have been reported in the literature.[27] Rates of tendon rupture following primary repair remain unfortunately high; historically rates of rupture were often cited between 4% and 30%.[28,29] However, with advances in technique, materials, and postoperative rehabilitation protocols, most recently reported rates of rupture approach 0% to 5%.[30,31] Multiple recent studies analyzing repair of Zone I and II lacerations report no ruptures in cohorts exceeding 50 to 100 patients.[32–34]

The most common reasons for rupture include an unplanned early loading of the repaired tendon, premature cessation of postoperative splinting, inadequate suture material, and aggressive early active range of motion protocols with insufficient repair strength.[28,35,36] In meta-analysis, age, gender, zone of injury, or surgical technique were not predictive of repair rupture.[6] The appropriate number of core strand sutures used for primary or revision repair remains a contentious issue. Increasing number of core strands confers greater strength at the cost of providing substantial bulk within an already confined fibro-osseous canal. Clinically, recent studies demonstrate noninferiority with fewer strand-repairs, yet most practitioners use a 4-core strand, locking technique.[37,38] In the pediatric population, often fewer core strands are used in the setting of anatomically smaller tendons.[39] *In vitro* studies demonstrate proportionally higher rupture force with the increasing number of corestrands.[35,40–42] Ruptures are more common with 2-strand repairs in the setting of early active range of motion protocols.[10]

In the event of rupture, most surgeons will opt for an immediate revision of the primary repair if technically feasible. However, alternative treatment options are available, depending on the zone of injury, digit involved, timing of rupture respective to initial repair, and patient-specific considerations. Excellent results can be achieved when repair is performed within 14 days of rupture.[43] In the event of delayed recognition of the rupture, or when attenuation at the site of repair exceeds 1 cm, the risk of quadrigia and excessive tensioning of transected tendon ends often precludes primary repair.[44] Similarly, when ruptures occur 4 to 6 weeks after the initial repair, primary repair is often unfeasible because of shortening and/or collapse of the sheath space, and secondary grafting is indicated. Other options for surgical management include 1-or-2 stage tendon grafting, arthrodesis of the distal interphalangeal joint (DIP) in the setting of an intact FDS, tenodesis if the distal FDP tendon provides sufficient length, or tendon transfers.

Preferred method of repair

In the setting of suspicion for rupture of a repaired tendon, operative exploration should be performed within the first 48 to 72 hours. On initial evaluation, the patient should be placed in dorsal blocking splint to prevent proximal excursion of the transected tendon. Provided there is minimal attenuation, proximal and distal ruptured tendon ends should be debrided to healthy tissue. A non-braided epitendinous suture, measuring 6 to 0, or 7 to 0, is performed to supplement a four-core strand suture repair. If rupture is limited to exclusively the FDS, repair is not necessary, and may exacerbate scar and adhesion formation. Should the degree of attenuation preclude attempted repair, staged reconstruction is indicated, as will be discussed later in this article (**Fig. 1**).

FLEXOR TENDON SCARRING

The most common complication following flexor tendon repair prompting revision surgery is adhesion formation, occurring in 4% to 10% of cases.[6,45] Reoperation occurs in approximately 6% of flexor tendon repairs and of these, tenolysis is the operation most performed and accounts for more than 50% of revision surgeries. Due to the unique anatomy of the flexor tendons and the surrounding fibro-osseous canal in Zone II, even marginal increases in bulk or slight anatomic changes can translate to significant limitations of tendon excursion. Factors that seem to impact adhesion/scar formation include the distribution and degree of trauma to the flexor tendon and surrounding sheath, tendon ischemia, duration of immobilization, and gapping at the tendon repair site.[25,46] Scar tissue forms in proportion to tissue trauma, and expectedly increases in the setting of crush injuries, highlighting the importance of atraumatic technique with any manipulation of the tendon directly during repair.[47] Factors such as age, gender, or zone of injury are not predictive of adhesion formation.[6]

Technically, the mitigation of adhesion formation is a difficult balance to attain due to opposing requirements of early mobilization, avoidance of excessive bulk within the tendon sheath, and minimization of gapping at the repair site. Early mobilization has become established as the preferred rehabilitation paradigm, although specifics of a universal and optimal regimen remain undefined. Concurrent injury to digital nerves portends a poor prognosis, lending credence to the belief that intact digital sensation is essential for adequate rehabilitation following tenolysis.[48] Clearly, early mobilization translates to improved biomechanical healing, and lower rates of subsequent tenolysis.[18,20,49–51] Some force applied across the repair site is essential for the promotion of proximal musculotendinous excursion; but excessive force can detrimentally induce gapping, and possibly induce rupture. Studies have shown

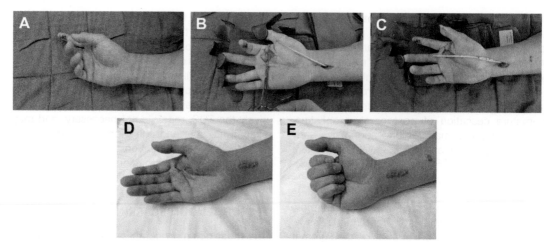

Fig. 1. *(A-E)* This patient suffered a rupture of a previous right index finger flexor digitorum profundus tendon repair in the palm. The flexor digitorum superficialis tendon was already absent from the trauma. *(A)* Posture of the finger before exploration. *(B)* Exploration reveals rupture of the flexor digitorum profundus proximal to zone II. *(C)* The ruptured tendon could not be repaired primarily; therefore, a palmaris longus tendon graft was used to lengthen the tendon. *(D)* Postoperative result with the finger in active extension. *(E)* Postoperative result with the finger in active flexion.

that gaps of as little as 3 mm can negatively impact the accrual of tendon strength as the tendon heals, predisposing to adhesion and scar formation.[52,53] Conversely, excursion of the tendon as little as 3 mm is sufficient to mitigate adhesion formation, though 6–9 mm is preferred to confer therapeutic benefit.[50,54]

Intraoperatively, the epitendinous and core sutures are used to mitigate adhesion formation. The use of controlled active motion protocols has gained popularity in concert with mechanically stronger repairs conferred using core sutures. Systematic review found that repairs using the modified Kessler technique were associated with a 57% lower likelihood of adhesion formation.[6] The use of an epitendinous suture has been shown to not only reduce the friction of flexor tendon repair site but also confers strength at the site of repair; ultimately, use of an epitendinous suture decreases rate of reoperation by 84%.[6,13,55,56] In the event of concurrent lacerations of FDP and FDS tendons, multiple studies document increased rates of tenolysis with repair of both tendons; consequently, many surgeons advocate for leaving the FDS unrepaired.[15,57] Thorough postoperative rehabilitation is essential to ensure minimal adhesion formation both after initial repair and following any revision tenolysis.[48]

After repair, mild adhesions can often be mitigated or remedied with rehabilitation; however, when excursion and range of motion have plateaued and passive motion significantly exceeds active, flexor tenolysis should be considered. Most surgeons will wait a minimum of 3 to 6 months before proceeding with operative intervention, allowing a sufficient duration for soft tissues to heal and reach "tissue equilibrium", whereby the skin is soft and pliable over the wound. Structural integrity of the repaired tendon and the surrounding sheath, supple joints and soft tissues, well-healed fractures in anatomic alignment, good muscle strength, and near normal passive range of motion are all prerequisites for the success of flexor tenolysis.[58–60] Due to distorted anatomy, the obliteration of natural tissue planes and scar formation, the surgery is technically difficult and should be approached with caution.[61] In the event of replanted or more extensively damaged digits, full passive range of motion may need to be achieved first with preliminary surgery consisting of extensor tenolysis and capsulotomy. The success of flexor tenolysis and the ability to regain active range of motion is predicated on the ability of a motivated patient to capitalize on the passive range of motion achieved by prior surgeries.

The use of wide-awake hand surgery has also positively impacted the availability and efficacy of tendon revision surgery. Historically, general anesthesia was preferred for any patient with tendon laceration due to the discomfort of a tourniquet, and thus required to expediently perform repair. More recently, with the injection of local anesthetic mixed with epinephrine, sufficient analgesia and vasoconstriction can be safely achieved to perform surgery in a bloodless field.[62,63] Contraindications for wide-awake surgery are relatively few; patients capable of following commands, with minimal anxiety or propensity to lose consciousness due to excessive vasovagal tone are appropriate candidates in most cases. The conscious patient is then able to participate in the active flexion and extension of the injured digit while on the table, facilitating appropriate tensioning of repair and assessment of unobstructed gliding.[64]

When performed adeptly, flexor tenolysis can significantly improve the function of injured patients. Multiple studies have demonstrated increases of greater than 50% in active range of motion in most of the digits operated on.[65–68] Complications including tendon rupture, protracted edema, pain, and injury to neurovascular structures, are possible and have been cited in the literature at a combined rate of 10% to 15%.[21,57,69]

Preferred Method of Tenolysis

Flexor tenolysis should be performed at least 3 to 6 months after definitive repair or reconstruction to allow maturity of the soft-tissue envelope ("tissue equilibrium"), healing of any associated fractures, and plateau in range of motion of injured digits despite continual hand therapy. In our institution, all tenolysis are performed in the operating room under the care of an anesthesiologist for reversible sedation, using a forearm tourniquet for the first part of the case. Anesthesia is performed using the injection of local anesthetic, namely lidocaine/bupivacaine with epinephrine, as well as reversible IV sedation, allowing the patient to perform active flexion in the operating room. The authors use any prior incisions, including healed scars from the inciting trauma, to gain access to the operative site. Should further exposure be necessary, prior incisions can be incorporated into a Brunauer, or mid-lateral incision to ensure adequate access.

Dissection should proceed from the uninjured/unaffected area with normal tendon to facilitate safe blunt dissection of the affected tendon. Preservation of the neurovascular bundles is paramount; they should be identified and safely retracted to avoid injury. A small window in a noncritical portion of the tendon sheath can be made to ensure access to the tendon proper. The borders of the tendons should be identified and released (**Fig. 2**A). A blunt elevator is then placed within the sheath and deep into the tendon to release adhesions along the tendon proximally and distally. Excursion of the FDP, if intact, takes precedence. If necessary, the FDS may need to be resected to optimize FDP motion. The status of the FDP tendon must be carefully determined

before the FDS is sacrificed. Full passive range of motion and joint motion is then assessed.

One trick is the use an Allis clamp to encircle the tendon atraumatically and then twirl the Allis clamp (**Fig. 2**B). This can provide proximal or distal distraction of the tendon without fear of rupturing the pulleys with upward tension. Then, sedation is turned off and the patient is asked to actively move the affected digits by making a composite fist (Video 1). Adequate active excursion and the integrity of pulleys with the absence of bowstringing must be achieved intraoperatively before closure. At this point, the patient is allowed immediate active and passive range of motion. If pain limits early participation with therapy, analgesic therapies, including an indwelling polyethylene catheter containing a local anesthetic, may be used.

Flexion Contracture

Despite optimal management, functional recovery can be hindered by flexion contracture in approximately 17% of repairs.[44] The etiology of joint contracture is variable and includes tendon bowstringing, injuries to the proximal interphalangeal (PIP) volar plate and surrounding stabilizing structures, and soft-tissue scar contracture. The most common cause of flexion contracture is excessive or suboptimal finger splinting. Following flexor tendon laceration repair, most surgeons and hand therapists recommend placement of the metacarpophalangeal (MCP) joints at approximately 90° of flexion, with the PIP and DIP joints fully extended. This position unloads the repair while keeping the collateral ligaments taut. Many contractures, if appreciated early, can be corrected nonoperatively. Adjuncts to splinting, including buddy taping and modifications to encourage the extension of the intrinsic mechanism, can be useful to correct early contracture. There are no established guidelines for surgical intervention. The same degree of contracture may be functionally limited in one patient, but tolerable to another. Therefore, indications for surgery are patient-specific and should balance operative risk and functional goals.

Preferred Method of Joint Release

Nonsurgical management includes early identification and splinting of the DIP and PIP joints in extension to relax the intrinsic mechanism and keep the collateral ligaments taut. If joint contractures persist, surgical joint release can occur 4 to 6 months after tendon repair depending on the patient's functional limitations and goals.[70] Intraoperatively, dissection should proceed systematically

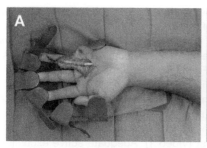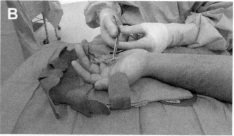

Fig. 2. *(A, B)* In this patient undergoing tenolysis of the left ring finger flexor tendon repair, *(A)* tenolysis is performed with the preservation of the A2 and A4 pulleys, *(B)* and an Allis clamp is used to atraumatically twirl the tendon, thereby mimicking pull.

and tissues should be released on a layer-by-layer basis. Release of PIP joint contracture is often performed in conjunction with flexor tenolysis. Soft tissue, including tethering scar tissue, should be released with care not to leave exposed tendon after the release. Most often, extension is limited by contracture of volar structures; as such the PIP is most often approached from the volar aspect of the joint. The volar plate and associated check-rein ligaments should be released as indicated. If insufficient, collateral ligaments should also be released to allow full extension at the PIP. One should be prepared for a soft tissue defect after contracture release. The patient should be counseled about the possible need for skin grafting or cross-finger flap coverage.

Salvage Flexor Tendon Reconstruction

Primary reconstruction using free-tendon grafts for Zone-II injuries was commonplace before the 1970s, and is currently performed less frequently given improved outcomes with direct repair and staged procedures in the event of rupture.[71] The use of tendon grafts in either 1 or 2 stages is often successful and yields promising clinical results.[71–74] Single staged grafting remains a viable option of repair in the event of segmental tendon loss, provided there remains an intact pulley system, supple joints, and grafting is performed in a clean wound bed with adequate soft-tissue coverage to ensure the early range of motion. Multiple graft donor sites are available and are broadly classified as either intra or extra-synovial. Extrasynovial tendon grafts consist of palmaris longus, plantaris, APL, and FCR among others. Intrasynovial tendon grafts consist of flexor digitorum superificialis, flexor digitorum longus (FDL), and extensor indicis proprius (EIP). No clinical studies have shown a superiority between the 2 groups, but extrasynovial tendons are thought to incite a greater inflammatory response, more adhesions, and resistance to gliding within the fibro-osseous

canal.[75–77] Technically, tenorrhaphy should be performed outside of the sheath proper, to avoid gliding of a bulky coaptation site. The injured proximal FDP should be used as the motor, although side-to-side coaptation to neighboring FDP slips or using the injured FDS are also feasible. Distally, the FDP remnant should be used for coaptation if of sufficient length of at least 7 to 11 mm. If of insufficient length, a pullout suture sewn over a button or bone anchor can be used to secure the distal pole of the graft.[78] Cadaveric studies demonstrate greater pull-out strength of the bone anchor.[79] Rarely, the plantaris tendon can be harvested en bloc with calcaneal bone, which can then be anchored into the injured digit via osteosynthesis.[80,81] Similar to direct repair, or the repair of a rupture, early range of motion rehabilitation is encouraged to achieve optimal results.[82]

In the event of an intact FDS but transected FDP, the residual strength of the superficialis is sufficient to confer flexion at the PIP. This may dilute the negative impact that compromise of DIP joint motion has on global hand function.[83] Deficiency of a moment arm across the distal interphalangeal joint can predispose to hyperextension of the joint with forceful pinch. Multiple salvage procedures can be performed for patients with exceptional dexterous requirements, including musicians and professions reliant on fine motor skills. For patients with sufficient distal FDP tendon, tenodesis is a viable option to confer excursion and stability of the DIP joint. Dynamic tenodesis procedures include the technique reported in Kahn and colleagues for which the distal stump is looped around the slips of the intact superficialis tendon, and sutured onto itself.[84] A modification of this technique using a split in the distal profundus tendon, with an intact proximal connection, has also been described. Despite technical feasibility and reported outcomes in cadaveric studies, there remains a paucity of clinical outcomes data regarding the utility of this technique.[85] If the proximal tendon cannot be retrieved, or the distal interphalangeal joint becomes grossly unstable, the patient can be offered DIP joint fusion to provide stability.

A two-staged approach to tendon reconstruction is recommended when injury results in sufficient tissue damage prompting excessive scarring, joint contracture, or an incompetent pulley apparatus.[86] Tendon repair or grafting placed in a violated fibro-osseous sheath is likely to be compromised by adhesions, obstruction, or bowstringing. Pioneering work in the 1960s and 1970s demonstrated not only the establishment of an organized cellular response to a gliding implant conducive to adequate tendon excursion, but also the revascularization of tendon grafts placed within that environment subsequent to the establishment of a fibro-osseous tunnel.[87,88] A staged reconstruction requires the initial establishment of an adequate pseudosheath via thorough exploration, reconstruction of the pulley apparatus with the concurrent release of any joint contracture, and finally placement of a prosthetic silicone rod. During the second stage, usually performed at an interval of 3 to 6 months thus allowing the consolidation of the pseudosheath around the prosthetic implant, the harvested graft is secured to the proximal motor, threaded through the newly formed pseudosheath, and secured distally.

Paneva-Holevich described a 2-staged method of reconstruction using a proximal tenorrhaphy between FDS and FDP tendons, providing a precoapted graft to be translated distally at the second stage.[89] This technique was later modified by Kessler in 1972, in which a silicone rod is placed within the fibro-osseous tunnel concurrently with the initial proximal coaptation.[90]

Good clinical outcomes can be achieved using staged reconstruction; rates of between 50% and 82% of patients achieve good to the excellent restoration of range of motion of injured digits as reported in the literature.[91–94] Unfortunately, a significant portion of patients undergoing staged tendon reconstruction, as high as 40%, will require tertiary surgery, including tenolysis.[95] Rates of complications following staged reconstruction are considerable, altogether as high as 41%, with ruptures occurring at a rate of 4% to 15%, and infection occurring in approximately 5% of cases.[96,97]

Preferred Method of Two-Staged Flexor Tendon Reconstruction

In the initial procedure, a regional anesthetic can be performed. The digit is approached either via a Brunauer or mid-lateral incision, again using prior traumatic lacerations, with avoidance of previously designed soft-tissue flaps (**Fig. 3**A). The mid-lateral incision may allow improved soft tissue coverage over the implant and subsequent tendon reconstruction. The residual scarred tendons are excised and the A2 & A4 pullies are examined (**Fig. 3**B). If the pulleys are missing, they can be reconstructed with the excised FDP or FDS tendon, wrapped around the phalanx, and sutured to the remnant edges of the pulley, all over the silicone rod sizer (**Fig. 3**C). The actual silicone rod is then passed through the pulleys, into and through the carpal tunnel, and into the forearm (**Fig. 3**D). Only the distal end of the silicone rod is coapted to the remaining FDP tendon; the proximal end of the silicone rod in the forearm is left free. Postoperative mobilization should be performed within 24 to 72 hours of the initial operation and continued until the next surgical stage to ensure joints remain a supple and full passive range of motion is achieved. A hand radiograph is always performed immediately before the second stage, just in case the silicone rod has broken free and has migrated proximally.

In the second stage, the patient receives a lower extremity regional anesthetic block in the anticipation of toe extensor tendon harvest. Toe extensor tendons are favored because they are longer than the palmaris longus and plantaris tendons. The patient is sedated and undergoes local anesthetic with epinephrine in the operative field applied to the distal finger and the distal forearm. The remainder of the finger and hand do not need to be incised or anesthetized.

A proximal forearm tourniquet is used for the first 30 minutes only, to avoid excessive muscle ischemia. The distal tendon/silicone rod site and the proximal silicone rod with its translucent pseudosheath are both identified. Once the free gliding of the silicone rod in situ is confirmed, it is then advisable to proceed with tendon grafting. Attention is then directed to the foot and leg, whereby the toe extensor harvest is performed (**Fig. 3**E). This is conducted via small horizontal incisions from the distal tendon, tracing proximally up the leg. Great care must be taken to anticipate branching junctura tendinae which make tendon stripping more difficult.

The graft is harvested and then brought to the operative field in the hand. It is tied to the distal end of the silicone rod and carefully passed into the sheath, gliding through the newly created tunnel until the proximal end is grasped in the forearm (**Fig. 3**F). Care is taken to make sure the tendon graft is controlled proximally and distally. The distal end of the tendon graft is secured to the distal tendon stump or directly to the distal

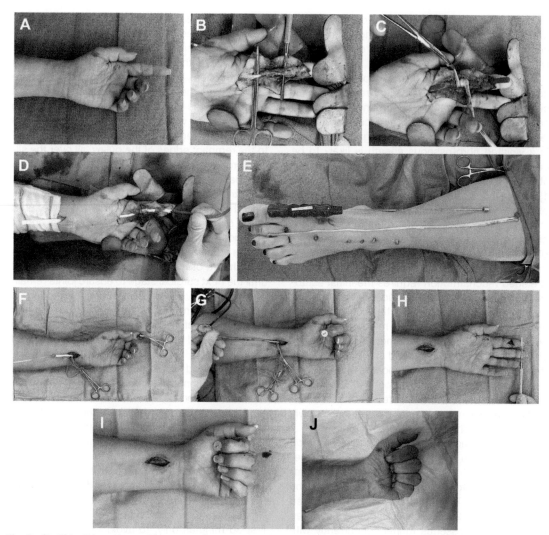

Fig. 3. *(A, B)* In this patient with a scarred, motionless finger after the previous attempt at flexor tendon repair, *(C)* the authors first reconstruct the A2 pully using the remnant flexor digitorum superficialis tendon. *(D)* Next, a Hunter rod is passed through the reconstructed pully while attached to a preliminary sizer. *(E)* In the second stage, the second toe extensor tendon is harvested. *(F)* The tendon graft is passed into the sheath by attaching it to the Hunter rod, which is then removed. *(G)* The distal juncture is tested by pulling on the tendon graft proximally. *(H)* Next, the tendon graft is woven into the index finger flexor digitorum profundus tendon proximally at the wrist, and tension is tested with the finger in extension to ensure it is not too tight. *(I)* Because this is conducted under wide-awake anesthesia, the patient can actively flex, thereby testing the tendon graft. *(J)* Final postoperative result with active finger flexion.

phalanx via a pull-out suture or suture anchor. The free proximal end of the tendon can be pulled to test that the finger flexes; this also tests the strength of the distal juncture (**Fig. 3**G). The free proximal end of the tendon graft is now passed through the selected proximal motor, most often the neighboring FDP tendon (**Fig. 3**H). At this point, the patient can be awakened from sedation to test if the proximal tendon motor unit is still working. Once the proximal motor tendon is chosen the tendon graft is passed into it via a

Pulvertaft weave. At least three passes are performed. Then, 1 or 2 sutures are placed to test the tension of the tendon graft. The patient should be able to immediately flex and extend the finger in the optimal arc (**Fig. 3**I). If not, the Pulvertaft weave can be loosened or tightened.

Wide-awake anesthesia has taken the guesswork out of flexor tendon grafting. These questions are answered by having the patient actively participate: (1) Are the repairs strong enough? (2) Is the tendon graft too loose or too tight? (3) Is there bowstringing? and (4) Is there residual tendon or scar in the palm causing a lumbrical plus deformity or quadriga? Finally, the wounds are closed, the patient is placed into a protective splint, and therapy is initiated 1 week after surgery (**Fig. 3**J).

SUMMARY

Despite improvements in our understanding of the physiology and biomechanics of tendon healing, functionally reliable repair of flexor tendon lacerations remains challenging and subject to complications including tendon rupture, adhesion formation, and joint contracture. Timely diagnosis and the adept performance of revision procedures such as primary tendon repair, flexor tenolysis, joint release, and two-staged flexor tendon reconstruction are essential in restoring good functional outcomes. In the past decade, advancements in operative technique and postoperative rehabilitation have helped to optimize functional results following the performance of these salvage procedures.

CLINICS CARE POINTS

- Complications in primary flexor tendon repair are common and include tendon rupture, adhesion formation, and joint contracture.

- Rupture of a repaired tendon should be addressed by early operative exploration, debridement, and revision with a four-core strand suture and nonbraided epitendinous suture.

- Adhesion formation may be mitigated with the use of epitendinous and core sutures, and early postoperative mobilization.

- Flexor tenolysis should be considered if the range of motion remains suboptimal (<180° of composite range of motion), progress has plateaued, and passive motion exceeds active motion.

- Wide-awake flexor tenolysis is preferred to allow the patient to perform active flexion in the operating room.

- Staged reconstruction is recommended when injury results in excessive scaring, joint contracture, or an incompetent pully apparatus.

DISCLOSURE

The authors have nothing to disclose.

SUPPLEMENTARY DATA

Supplementary data related to this article can be found online at https://doi.org/10.1016/j.hcl.2022.08.021.

REFERENCES

1. de Jong JP, Nguyen JT, Sonnema AJM, et al. The Incidence of Acute Traumatic Tendon Injuries in the Hand and Wrist: A 10-Year Population-based Study. Clin Orthop Surg 2014;6(2):196–202.
2. Chan TK, Ho CO, Lee WK, et al. Functional outcome of the hand following flexor tendon repair at the "no man's land. J Orthop Surg Hong Kong 2006;14(2):178–83.
3. O'Connell SJ, Moore MM, Strickland JW, et al. Results of zone I and zone II flexor tendon repairs in children. J Hand Surg 1994;19(1):48–52.
4. Sikora S, Lai M, Arneja JS. Pediatric flexor tendon injuries: A 10-year outcome analysis. Can J Plast Surg J Can Chir Plast 2013;21(3):181–5.
5. Bunnell S. Surgery of the Hand. 1st edition.; 1944.
6. Dy CJ, Hernandez-Soria A, Ma Y, et al. Complications after flexor tendon repair: a systematic review and meta-analysis. J Hand Surg 2012;37(3):543–51.e1.
7. Moriya K, Yoshizu T, Tsubokawa N, et al. Incidence of tenolysis and features of adhesions in the digital flexor tendons after multi-strand repair and early active motion. J Hand Surg Eur 2019;44(4):354–60.
8. Beredjiklian PK. Biologic aspects of flexor tendon laceration and repair. ' Bone Joint Surg Am 2003;85(3):539–50.
9. Chartier C, ElHawary H, Baradaran A, et al. Tendon: Principles of Healing and Repair. Semin Plast Surg 2021;35(3):211–5.
10. Xu H, Huang X, Guo Z, et al. Outcome of Surgical Repair and Rehabilitation of Flexor Tendon Injuries in Zone II of the Hand: Systematic Review and Meta-Analysis. J Hand Surg 2022;S0363-5023(21):755–63. Published online February 4.
11. Zhao C, Amadio PC, Zobitz ME, et al. Gliding characteristics of tendon repair in canine flexor digitorum profundus tendons. J Orthop Res Off Publ Orthop Res Soc 2001;19(4):580–6.
12. Zhao C, Amadio PC, Paillard P, et al. Digital resistance and tendon strength during the first week after flexor digitorum profundus tendon repair in a canine model in vivo. J Bone Joint Surg Am 2004;86(2):320–7.
13. Moriya T, Zhao C, An KN, et al. The Effect of Epitendinous Suture Technique on Gliding Resistance During Cyclic Motion After Flexor Tendon Repair: A Cadaveric Study. J Hand Surg 2010;35(4):552–8.
14. Tang JB. Release of the A4 Pulley to Facilitate Zone II Flexor Tendon Repair. J Hand Surg 2014;39(11):2300–7.

15. Tang JB. Recent evolutions in flexor tendon repairs and rehabilitation. J Hand Surg Eur 2018;43(5):469–73.

16. Moriya K, Yoshizu T, Tsubokawa N, et al. Clinical results of releasing the entire A2 pulley after flexor tendon repair in zone 2C. J Hand Surg Eur 2016;41(8):822–8.

17. Peters SE, Jha B, Ross M. Rehabilitation following surgery for flexor tendon injuries of the hand. Cochrane Database Syst Rev 2021;1:CD012479.

18. Lister GD, Kleinert HE, Kutz JE, et al. Primary flexor tendon repair followed by immediate controlled mobilization. J Hand Surg 1977;2(6):441–51.

19. Small JO, Brennen MD, Colville J. Early active mobilisation following flexor tendon repair in zone 2. J Hand Surg Edinb Scotl 1989;14(4):383–91.

20. Woo SLY, Gelberman RH, Cobb NG, et al. The Importance of Controlled Passive Mobilization on Flexor Tendon Healing: A Biomechanical Study. Acta Orthop Scand 1981;52(6):615–22.

21. Lilly SI, Messer TM. Complications after treatment of flexor tendon injuries. J Am Acad Orthop Surg 2006;14(7):387–96.

22. Maloon S, de V de Beer J, Opitz M, et al. Acute flexor tendon sheath infections. J Hand Surg 1990;15(3):474–7.

23. Stone JF, Davidson JS. The role of antibiotics and timing of repair in flexor tendon injuries of the hand. Ann Plast Surg 1998;40(1):7–13.

24. Glass KD. Factors related to the resolution of treated hand infections. J Hand Surg 1982;7(4):388–94.

25. Legrand A, Kaufman Y, Long C, et al. Molecular Biology of Flexor Tendon Healing in Relation to Reduction of Tendon Adhesions. J Hand Surg 2017;42(9):722–6.

26. Wong JKF, Lui YH, Kapacee Z, et al. The Cellular Biology of Flexor Tendon Adhesion Formation. Am J Pathol 2009;175(5):1938–51.

27. Eshman SJ, Posner MA, Green SM, et al. Intratendinous rupture of a flexor tendon graft many years after staged reconstruction: A report of three cases. J Hand Surg 2000;25(6):1135–9.

28. Harris SB, Harris D, Foster AJ, et al. The aetiology of acute rupture of flexor tendon repairs in zones 1 and 2 of the fingers during early mobilization. J Hand Surg Edinb Scotl 1999;24(3):275–80.

29. Baktir A, Türk CY, Kabak S, et al. Flexor tendon repair in zone 2 followed by early active mobilization. J Hand Surg Edinb Scotl 1996;21(5):624–8.

30. Hoffmann GL, Büchler U, Vögelin E. Clinical results of flexor tendon repair in zone II using a six-strand double-loop technique compared with a two-strand technique. J Hand Surg Eur 2008;33(4):418–23.

31. Khor WS, Langer MF, Wong R, et al. Improving Outcomes in Tendon Repair: A Critical Look at the Evidence for Flexor Tendon Repair and Rehabilitation. Plast Reconstr Surg 2016;138(6):1045e–58e.

32. Fs F, Vs K, Ij G, et al. Primary flexor tendon repair in zones 1 and 2: early passive mobilization versus controlled active motion. J Hand Surg 2014;39(7). https://doi.org/10.1016/j.jhsa.2014.03.025.

33. Giesen T, Calcagni M, Elliot D. Primary Flexor Tendon Repair with Early Active Motion: Experience in Europe. Hand Clin 2017;33(3):465–72.

34. Tang JB, Zhou X, Pan ZJ, et al. Strong Digital Flexor Tendon Repair, Extension-Flexion Test, and Early Active Flexion: Experience in 300 Tendons. Hand Clin 2017;33(3):455–63.

35. Wagner WF, Carroll C, Strickland JW, et al. A biomechanical comparison of techniques of flexor tendon repair. J Hand Surg 1994;19(6):979–83.

36. Pulos N, Bozentka DJ. Management of complications of flexor tendon injuries. Hand Clin 2015;31(2):293–9.

37. Hardwicke JT, Tan JJ, Foster MA, et al. A systematic review of 2-strand versus multistrand core suture techniques and functional outcome after digital flexor tendon repair. J Hand Surg 2014;39(4):686–95. e2.

38. Shaharan S, Bage T, Ibrahim N, et al. Rupture Rates Between 2-Strand and 4-Strand Flexor Tendon Repairs: Is Less More? Ann Plast Surg 2020;84(1):43–6.

39. Cooper L, Khor W, Burr N, et al. Flexor tendon repairs in children: Outcomes from a specialist tertiary centre. J Plast Reconstr Aesthet Surg 2015;68(5):717–23.

40. Lawrence TM, Woodruff MJ, Aladin A, et al. An assessment of the tensile properties and technical difficulties of two- and four-strand flexor tendon repairs. J Hand Surg Br Eur 2005;30(3):294–7.

41. Barrie KA, Wolfe SW, Shean C, et al. A biomechanical comparison of multistrand flexor tendon repairs using an in situ testing model. J Hand Surg 2000;25(3):499–506.

42. Thurman RT, Trumble TE, Hanel DP, et al. Two-, four-, and six-strand zone II flexor tendon repairs: an in situ biomechanical comparison using a cadaver model. J Hand Surg 1998;23(2):261–5.

43. Allen BN, Frykman GK, Unsell RS, et al. Ruptured flexor tendon tenorrhaphies in zone II: repair and rehabilitation. J Hand Surg 1987;12(1):18–21.

44. Taras JS, Gray RM, Culp RW. COMPLICATIONS OF FLEXOR TENDON INJURIES. Hand Clin 1994;10(1):93–109.

45. Tang JB. Clinical outcomes associated with flexor tendon repair. Hand Clin 2005;21(2):199–210.

46. Matthews P, Richards H. Factors in the adherence of flexor tendon after repair: an experimental study in the rabbit. J Bone Joint Surg Br 1976;58(2):230–6.

47. Feehan LM, Beauchene JG. Early tensile properties of healing chicken flexor tendons: early controlled passive motion versus postoperative immobilization. J Hand Surg 1990;15(1):63–8.

48. Diehm YF, Haug V, Thomé J, et al. The Impact of Digital Nerve Injury on the Outcome of Flexor Tendon Tenolysis: A Retrospective Case-Control Study. Ann Plast Surg 2021;87(5):514–7.

49. Hitchcock TF, Light TR, Bunch WH, et al. The effect of immediate constrained digital motion on the strength of flexor tendon repairs in chickens. J Hand Surg 1987;12(4):590–5.

50. DURAN R. A preliminary report in the use of controlled passive motion following flexor tendon repair in zones II and III. J Hand Surg 1976;1:79.

51. Aoki M, Kubota H, Pruitt DL, et al. Biomechanical and histologic characteristics of canine flexor tendon repair using early postoperative mobilization. J Hand Surg 1997;22(1):107–14.

52. Gelberman RH, Boyer MI, Brodt MD, et al. The effect of gap formation at the repair site on the strength and excursion of intrasynovial flexor tendons. An experimental study on the early stages of tendon-healing in dogs. J Bone Joint Surg Am 1999;81(7):975–82.

53. Silfverskiöld KL, May EJ. Gap formation after flexor tendon repair in zone II. Results with a new controlled motion programme. Scand J Plast Reconstr Surg Hand Surg 1993;27(4):263–8.

54. Silfverskiöld KL, May EJ, Törnvall AH. Tendon excursions after flexor tendon repair in zone. II: Results with a new controlled-motion program. J Hand Surg 1993;18(3):403–10.

55. Xu NM, Brown PJ, Plate JF, et al. Fibrin glue augmentation for flexor tendon repair increases friction compared with epitendinous suture. J Hand Surg 2013;38(12):2329–34.

56. Diao E, Hariharan JS, Soejima O, et al. Effect of peripheral suture depth on strength of tendon repairs. J Hand Surg 1996;21(2):234–9.

57. Civan O, Gürsoy MK, Cavit A, et al. Tenolysis rate after zone 2 flexor tendon repairs. Jt Dis Relat Surg 2020;31(2):281–5.

58. Fetrow KO. Tenolysis in the hand and wrist. A clinical evaluation of two hundred and twenty flexor and extensor tenolyses. J Bone Joint Surg Am 1967;49(4):667–85.

59. Whitaker JH, Strickland JW, Ellis RK. The role of flexor tenolysis in the palm and digits. J Hand Surg 1977;2(6):462–70.

60. Azari KK, Meals RA. Flexor tenolysis. Hand Clin 2005;21(2):211–7.

61. Strickland JW. Flexor Tenolysis. Hand Clin 1985;1(1):121–32.

62. Thomson CJ, Lalonde DH, Denkler KA, et al. A critical look at the evidence for and against elective epinephrine use in the finger. Plast Reconstr Surg 2007;119(1):260–6.

63. Lalonde DH. Wide-Awake Flexor Tendon Repair. Plast Reconstr Surg 2009;123(2):623–5.

64. Gao LL, Chang J. Wide Awake Secondary Tendon Reconstruction. Hand Clin 2019;35(1):35–41.

65. Foucher G, Lenoble E, Ben Youssef K, et al. A postoperative regime after digital flexor tenolysis. A series of 72 patients. J Hand Surg Edinb Scotl 1993;18(1):35–40.

66. Hahn P, Krimmer H, Müller L, et al. [Outcome of flexor tenolysis after injury in zone 2]. Handchir Mikrochir Plast Chir Organ Deutschsprachigen Arbeitsgemeinschaft Handchir Organ Deutschsprachigen Arbeitsgemeinschaft Mikrochir Peripher Nerven Gefasse Organ V 1996;28(4):198–203.

67. Eggli S, Dietsche A, Eggli S, et al. Tenolysis after combined digital injuries in zone II. Ann Plast Surg 2005;55(3):266–71.

68. Jupiter JB, Pess GM, Bour CJ. Results of flexor tendon tenolysis after replantation in the hand. J Hand Surg 1989;14(1):35–44.

69. Breton A, Jager T, Dap F, et al. Effectiveness of flexor tenolysis in zone II: A retrospective series of 40 patients at 3 months postoperatively. Chir Main 2015;34(3):126–33.

70. Moore T, Anderson B, Seiler JG. Flexor tendon reconstruction. J Hand Surg 2010;35(6):1025–30.

71. Boyes JH, Stark HH. Flexor-Tendon Grafts in the Fingers and Thumb: A STUDY OF FACTORS INFLUENCING RESULTS IN 1000 CASES. JBJS 1971;53(7):1332–42.

72. Pulvertaft RG. The Treatment of Profundus Division by Free Tendon Graft. JBJS 1960;42(8):1363–80.

73. McClinton MA, Curtis RM, Wilgis EFS. One hundred tendon grafts for isolated flexor digitorum profundus injuries. J Hand Surg 1982;7(3):224–9.

74. Sakellarides HT, Papadopoulos G. Surgical treatment of the divided flexor digitorum profundus tendon in zone 2, delayed more than 6 weeks, by tendon grafting in 50 cases. J Hand Surg Edinb Scotl 1996;21(1):63–6.

75. Uchiyama S, Amadio PC, Ishikawa J, et al. Boundary lubrication between the tendon and the pulley in the finger. J Bone Joint Surg Am 1997;79(2):213–8.

76. Nishida J, Amadio PC, Bettinger PC, et al. Excursion properties of tendon graft sources: interaction between tendon and A2 pulley. J Hand Surg 1998;23(2):274–8.

77. Leversedge FJ, Zelouf D, Williams C, et al. Flexor tendon grafting to the hand: an assessment of the intrasynovial donor tendon-A preliminary single-cohort study. J Hand Surg 2000;25(4):721–30.

78. Kang N, Marsh D, Dewar D. The morbidity of the button-over-nail technique for zone 1 flexor tendon repairs. Should we still be using this technique? J Hand Surg Eur 2008;33(5):566–70.

79. Brustein M, Pellegrini J, Choueka J, et al. Bone suture anchors versus the pullout button for repair of distal profundus tendon injuries: a comparison of strength in human cadaveric hands. J Hand Surg 2001;26(3):489–96.

80. Bertelli JA, Santos MA, Kechele PR, et al. Flexor tendon grafting using a plantaris tendon with a

fragment of attached bone for fixation to the distal phalanx: a preliminary cohort study. J Hand Surg 2007;32(10):1543–8.

81. Dos Santos MA, Bertelli JA, Kechele PR, et al. Anatomical study of the plantaris tendon: reliability as a tendo-osseous graft. Surg Radiol Anat SRA 2009;31(1):59–61.

82. Clancy SP, Mass DP. Current flexor and extensor tendon motion regimens: a summary. Hand Clin 2013;29(2):295–309.

83. Moiemen NS, Elliot D. Primary flexor tendon repair in zone 1. J Hand Surg Br Eur 2000;25(1):78–84.

84. Kahn S. A dynamic tenodesis of the distal interphalangeal joint, for use after severance of the profundus alone. Plast Reconstr Surg 1973;51(5):536–40.

85. Pritsch T, Sammer DM. Tenodesis for restoration of distal interphalangeal joint flexion in unrepairable flexor digitorum profundus injuries. J Hand Surg 2014;39(1):19–23.

86. Hunter JM, Salisbury RE. Flexor-tendon reconstruction in severely damaged hands. A two-stage procedure using a silicone-dacron reinforced gliding prosthesis prior to tendon grafting. J Bone Joint Surg Am 1971;53(5):829–58.

87. Hunter JM, Subin D, Minkow F, et al. Sheath formation in response to limited active gliding implants (animals). J Biomed Mater Res 1974;8(3):163–73.

88. Urbaniak JR, Bright DS, Gill LH, et al. Vascularization and the Gliding Mechanism of Free Flexor-Tendon Grafts Inserted by the Silicone-Rod Method. JBJS 1974;56(3):473–82.

89. Paneva-Holevich E. Two-stage tenoplasty in injury of the flexor tendons of the hand. J Bone Joint Surg Am 1969;51(1):21–32.

90. Kessler FB. Use of a pedicled tendon transfer with a silicone rod in complicated secondary flexor tendon repairs. Plast Reconstr Surg 1972;49(4):439–43.

91. Paneva-Holevich E. Two-stage reconstruction of the flexor tendons. Int Orthop 1982;6(2):133–8.

92. Alnot JY, Mouton P, Bisson P. [Longstanding flexor tendon lesions treated by two-stage tendon graft]. Ann Chir Main Memb Superieur Organe Off Soc Chir Main Ann Hand Up Limb Surg 1996;15(1):25–35.

93. Beris AE, Darlis NA, Korompilias AV, et al. Two-stage flexor tendon reconstruction in zone II using a silicone rod and a pedicled intrasynovial graft. J Hand Surg 2003;28(4):652–60.

94. Sun S, Ding Y, Ma B, et al. Two-stage flexor tendon reconstruction in zone II using Hunter's technique. Orthopedics 2010;33(12):880.

95. Finsen V. Two-stage grafting of digital flexor tendons: a review of 43 patients after 3 to 15 years. Scand J Plast Reconstr Surg Hand Surg 2003;37(3):159–62.

96. Wehbé MA, Mawr B, Hunter JM, et al. Two-stage flexor-tendon reconstruction. Ten-year experience. JBJS 1986;68(5):752–63.

97. Coyle MP, Leddy TP, Leddy JP. Staged flexor tendon reconstruction fingertip to palm. J Hand Surg 2002;27(4):581–5.

Hand Flexor Tendon Repair
From Biology to Surgery and Rehabilitation

Cristian Aletto, MD[a,b,*], Rocco Aicale, MD[a,b], Francesco Oliva, MD[a,b],
Nicola Maffulli, MD, MS, PhD, FRCS (Orth)[a,b,c,d]

KEYWORDS

• Hand • Tendon • Flexor • Hand rehabilitation • Tendon biology

KEY POINTS

• Hand flexor tendons are collagen I based tissues covered by synovial sheaths which reduce mechanical stress.
• The volar aspect of the hand is divided in V zone, they are important for treatment and rehabilitation.
• The process of tendon healing must be considered before and after surgery to allow tissue reconstruction and limit the amount of fibrosis in the surrounding tissues.
• Early mobilisation reduces adhesion formation and improves quality of tendon healing.
• Adjuvant therapies have been studied to prevent the adhesiogenic nature of tendon repair.

INTRODUCTION

Before the 1960s, tendon repairs of the hand were rarely performed because of the universally poor outcomes, especially when the lacerations were in zone II. In the last few years, research has focused on different suture configurations or number of core sutures to maximize the strength of tendon repair, and on postoperative rehabilitation protocols to maximize outcomes.[1]

Tendon repair aims to achieve enough tendon strength to allow early motion, prevent adhesions within the tendon sheath, and to restore the normal range of motion (ROM) and function of the injured finger. Tendons can tolerate compression forces and shear forces, they incorporate sesamoid bones, and they act as a buffer by absorbing external forces to limit muscle damage.

Basic Anatomy of the Flexor Tendons of the Hand

Tendons are collagen-based tissues that connect muscle to bone and are primarily composed of type I collagen, whereas the surrounding endotenon and epitenon are primarily composed of type III collagen.[2]

Anatomically organized according to a precise hierarchical scheme, the cellular components of tendons are made in part of cells called tenocytes (TCs) and tenoblasts (which represent 90% to 95% of the cellular elements), and in part of long bundles of type I collagen with a small quantity of other types of collagen, proteoglycans with hydrophilics chains of glycosaminglycans (GAGs), glycoproteins and neurovascular structures.[3]

The extracellular matrix (ECM) helps with gliding between collagen fibrils and provides functional

[a] Department of Musculoskeletal Disorders, Faculty of Medicine and Surgery, University of Salerno, Baronissi 84084, Italy; [b] Clinica Ortopedica, Ospedale San Giovanni di Dio e Ruggi D'Aragona, Salerno 84131, Italy; [c] Queen Mary University of London, Barts and the London School of Medicine and Dentistry, Centre for Sports and Exercise Medicine, Mile End Hospital, 275 Bancroft Road, London E1 4DG, England; [d] Keele University, Faculty of Medicine, School of Pharmacy and Bioengineering, Guy Hilton Research Centre, Thornburrow Drive, Hartshill, Stoke-on-Trent ST4 7QB, UK
* Corresponding author. Department of Musculoskeletal Disorders, Faculty of Medicine and Surgery, University of Salerno, Baronissi 84084, Italy.
E-mail address: cris.aletto28@gmail.com

Hand Clin 39 (2023) 215–225
https://doi.org/10.1016/j.hcl.2022.12.001

hand.theclinics.com

stability to the fibers. Proteoglycans are the main molecules responsible for tendon visco-elasticity.[4] To facilitate sliding and produce a channel for blood vessels, a very thin structure of connective tissue called "endotenon" is interposed between fibers.[5] The endotenon continues in a sheet of connective-tissue, the "epitenon," which externally surrounds the tendon, containing the vascular, lymphatic, and nerve supplies of the tendon.[5]

At the myotendinous junction, tendinous collagen fibrils are inserted into deep recesses formed by myocyte processes, allowing the tension produced by intracellular contractile proteins of muscle fibers to be transmitted to the collagen fibrils.[6] This complex architecture reduces the tensile stress exerted on a tendon during muscle contraction. However, this junction still remains the weakest point of the muscle-tendon unit.[7]

The osteotendinous junction (OTJ) is composed of four zones: tendon, fibrocartilage, mineralized fibrocartilage, and bone.[8] The specialized structure of the OTJ prevents collagen or fiber bending, fraying, shearing, and failure.[9,10]

Synovial tendon sheaths are found in the areas subjected to increased mechanical stress, such as the tendons of the hand and foot, where efficient lubrication is required. Synovial sheaths consist of an outer fibrotic sheath and an inner synovial sheath, formed by thin visceral and parietal sheets.[11] The inner synovial sheath invests the tendon body, resulting as an ultrafiltration membrane to produce synovial fluid. The fibrous sheath forms condensations, the "pulleys," which act as fulcrums to aid tendon function.[12] The flexor tendon sheath starts with the first annular pulley, or A1; there are a total of five annular pulleys (A1 to A5) and three cruciate pulleys (C1–C3). The A2 and A4 pulleys are the most important biomechanically for digital motion and power. The cruciate pulleys are collapsible and flexible, allowing digital flexion without deformation of the pulley system. In addition, the oblique pulley can prevent bowstringing of the flexor pollicis longus[13]

Flexor digitorum profundus (FDP) and flexor digitorum superficialis (FDS) tendons receive dual nutritional supply by vascular perfusion and synovial diffusion.[14,15] Each tendon receives vascular supply by vincula, classified as longus and brevis. Commonly, a vinculum inserts on the dorsal aspect of the tendon, creating a richer blood supply on the same side. For this reason, vincula are important in the repair of injured tendons, and surgeons must be careful not to damage any of them to avoid decreasing the already limited blood supply.[14]

The hand has been divided in five anatomic zones, which include the region from the FDS insertion to the FDP tendon (zone I), the proximal aspect of the A1 pulley to the FDS insertion (zone II), the distal transverse aspect of the carpal ligament to the A1 pulley (zone III), the carpal tunnel (zone IV), and the proximal border of the transverse carpal ligament to the musculotendinous junction in the proximal forearm (zone V)[16] (**Fig. 1**).

The process of tendon healing should coordinate tissue reconstruction and limit the amount of fibrosis in the surrounding tissues. The initial healing of flexor tendons is characterized by three separate stages: inflammatory, fibroblastic or reparative, and remodeling.[17]

Starting during the first week after injury, blood vessels and tendon sheath form a clot at the injury site involving vasodilators and pro-inflammatory cells, which are able to remove necrotic tissue, fibrin clot, and cellular debris through phagocytosis. During the third week after injury, the fibroblastic stage begins: fibroblasts rapidly proliferate and synthetize immature collagen with the production of ECM. The initial collagen is type III, weaker than compared with type I.

After 6 to 8 weeks, the remodeling stage starts. Type I collagen fibers are reorganized in a longitudinal fashion along the tendon long axis, and fibrils begin crosslinked, increasing the strength of the complex. However, the end result will never completely restore the normal native tendon anatomy.[17]

Biomechanics of Healing

At present, it is not possible to fully restore the normal biomechanical properties of native tendon. After surgical fixation, tendons undergo a decrease in their tension strength, and only during the remodeling stage this starts to increase, together with the progressive replacement of type I collagen.[2]

Controlled early active mobilization (EAM) of the repaired flexor finger tendons increases the stresses across the repair site. If the stress is below the level for repair failure, collagen deposition across the repair site is increased, decreasing adhesions between the tendon and its surrounding sheath. This is the basis for early mobilization immediately after surgical repair of the tendon.

Zone and Type of Flexor Tendon Injuries

Zone I

Zone I lies between the FDP tendon to the insertion of the FDS tendon. Commonly, injuries in this area are laceration or avulsion, and occur in young

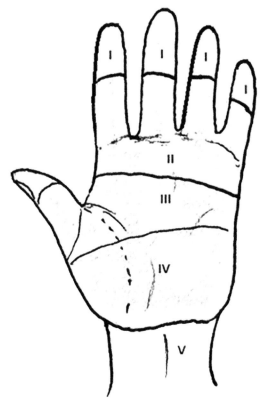

Fig. 1. Flexor system zones. I: distal to the flexor digitorum superficialis insertion; II: from the proximal aspect of the A1 pulley to the insertion of the flexor digitorum superficialis; III: the distal transverse aspect of the carpal ligament to the A1 pulley; IV: the carpal tunnel; and V: proximal to the carpal tunnel.

adults. Leddy and Packer[18] classified subtypes of zone I avulsion injuries.

Type I involves retraction of the proximal stump of the FDP to the palm. Both vincula are disrupted, and the tendon remains devoid of nutrition. In general, this type of trauma has the worst prognosis.

Type II avulsions, injured tendon retracts to the level of the proximal interphalangeal (PIP) joint. Surgical correction is less urgent because there is less potential for contracture and necrosis.

Type III, avulsions are characterized by large bony fragments that prevent the retraction over the A4 pulley.

Type IV Injuries are Challenging Injuries, Involving Fracture and Avulsion of the FDP Tendon from the Fracture Fragment.[19]

Zone II

Zone II runs from the proximal aspect of the A1 pulley to the insertion of the FDS. Injuries in this zone are particularly difficult to manage resulting in poor outcomes due to poor vascular supply, an increased risk of adhesions, the need to

accommodate two tendons in a tight fibro-osseous tunnel, catching and triggering the repaired tendon under the A2 pulley.[20]

Zone III

It includes the area from the distal transverse aspect of the carpal ligament to the A1 pulley. Given the absence of a sheath, injuries in this zone often have a good prognosis. A carpal tunnel release can be required in the proximal zone III to facilitate retrieval of the damaged tendon.[21]

Zone IV

It is the carpal tunnel zone, and tendon injuries are typically laceration. Pure tendon injuries are rare given the protective effect of the flexor retinaculum; however, injuries may involve the median or ulnar nerve. Treatment includes the release of the transverse carpal ligament and direct tendon repair.[22]

Zone V

Zone V goes from the proximal border of the transverse carpal ligament and ends at the musculotendinous junction in the proximal forearm. Injuries occur concurrently with nerve or vascular trauma, and management consists of at least four core sutures and epitendinous repair.[23]

SURGICAL TECHNIQUES

Improvements in suture design and rehabilitation methods have made primary hand flexor tendon repair the preferred operative treatment of acute laceration.

Primary tendon repair is defined as the repair performed within 24h from time of injury; a *delayed primary repair* is performed between 24h and 10 days; a repair after 10 to 14 days is called *secondary repair;* after 4 weeks, it is called *late secondary repair.*

The accurate coaptation of the tendon stumps allows early postoperative rehabilitation, promoting tendon gliding, inhibiting peritendinous adhesions formation, and restoring normal finger ROM.[24]

Principles of Flexor Tendon Repair

The two basic components of the suture techniques are the core suture and the epitendinous suture. A core suture is a suture that passes through the tendon and grasps it, traversing across the tendon. The final knot is buried within the repair site or lies on its surface. The widely used core suture configurations are the Kessler's and the modified Kessler's suture. They have two strands of sutures running across the repair site with an added "epitendinous" suture running all around the tendon surface.

The modified Kessler has only one final knot in the core suture as opposed to the original Kessler suture which has 2 knots. More complex configurations (**Fig. 2**) such as the Tajima, the Strickland, the cruciate, the Becker and the Savage, offer great tensile strength,[25] but do not improve outcomes and are associated with a higher risk of adhesions.[17] However, a two-strand repair allows only for passive mobilization protocols and cannot withstand active mobilization regimens (**Fig. 3**).

Biomechanically, the two-strand repair techniques show increased gap formation whereas the six-strand repair techniques increase tensile strength. Multiple strands increase tendon damage inducing ischemia and compromising intrinsic healing, and at the same time, they increase the bulk of the repaired site. A looped, four-strand modified Kessler can be a possible solution to minimize the friction between the tendon and its sheath while maintaining adequate strength to provide a wide margin of safety during physiotherapy.[24] The epitendinous suture is applied circumferentially and deeply around the tendon repair site; it makes the repair site smooth and adds strength to the repair. Strickland[13] outlined the principles of flexor tendon repair: they include easy placement of sutures in the tendon, secure suture knots, smooth juncture of the tendon ends, minimal gapping at the repair site, minimal interference with tendon vascularity, and sufficient strength throughout healing to allow early tendon motion. Repair strength is influenced by the caliber of the suture material used, the number of core sutures, and the purchase length of the suture.[26] An epitendinous suture may improve the biomechanical strength of the tendon repair, minimizing the gap, and reducing the cross-sectional area, which subsequently decreases gliding friction. Minimization of gap formation is essential in zone II injuries; indeed, 3 mm or more of gap formation has been associated with adhesions, increased gliding resistance, and decreased strength of the repair site.[27] Knots are the weakest component of the construct, and most failures occur here. Internal knots decrease the strength of the suture when compared with the external knots at day zero of repair, but, after 6 weeks, there is no difference in tensile strength. However, internal knots seem to stimulate tendon healing.[28]

Repair of Tendon Injuries in Zone I

Injuries in zone 1 typically involve two kinds of injuries: distal FDP tendon laceration to the insertion of the FDS tendon, or FDP avulsion from its insertion at the base of the distal phalanx.

Acute zone I injuries typically need to be treated to prevent hyperextension of the distal interphalangeal (DIP) joint, a condition that could decrease grip and pinch strength.[29]

When a tendon is lacerated, the distal tendon stump should be considered. If the distal tendon stump is less than 1 cm long, FDP tendon advancement and primary repair to bone should be performed. Tendon-to-bone repair can be obtained through traditional pull-out suture methods or internal suture methods. When the distal tendon stump is longer than 1 cm, primary tenorrhaphy is preferred.[30]

If FDP tendon is avulsed, four types of avulsions can occur according to Leddy and Packer classification. Type I avulsions require urgent surgical repair, whereas in type II avulsions surgery can be delayed up to 6 weeks after injury. In type III, proximal tendon retraction beyond the A4 pulley presents just the proximal migration of the fragment, and the fracture must be fixed with a Kirschner wire or a small screw. A type IV injury is defined as a fracture and avulsion of the FDP tendon from the fracture fragment. At first, the fracture is addressed. Afterward, the tendon, located within the tendon sheath or within the palm, is advanced and fixed to the distal phalanx. In some cases, with a small fracture fragment, the bone may be excised, and tendon can be advanced and sutured into the distal phalanx. Generally, a type IV injury is more severe and may be associated with a less optimal outcome.[31] When injuries are reconstructed, loss of DIPJ motion

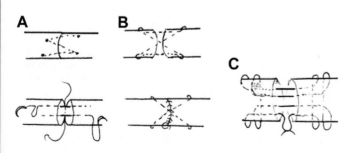

Fig. 2. Combinations of core sutures that can be used for flexor tendon repair, that is, (*A*) four-, (*B*) six-, and (*C*) eight-strand core configurations.

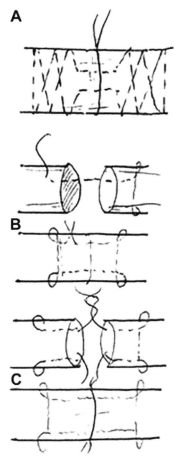

Fig. 3. Kessler suture and its modifications are the most studied and used due to its easy configuration. (*A*) Bunnell suture configuration (*B*) Kessler grasping suture configuration (*C*) Kessler-Tajima suture configuration.

is common, and in case of pain or symptomatic discomfort, they can be managed with a DIPJ arthrodesis.[32]

Repair of Zone 2 Tendon Injuries

Zone 2 is also called by Bunnell "no man's land," because, in the World War I the term indicated such a tract of battled-over land over which neither of the opposing armies has established control and where no man should trespass.[33] So, it was suggested that no man should attempt to repair tendon injuries in this zone. At present, core sutures provide an end-to-end tendons coaptation strong enough to achieve good clinical outcomes and early digital mobilization.

The FDP tendon within zones 1 and 2 is ideal for double-strand or four-strand core suture placement.

For smaller tendons, a four-strand modified Kessler suture is preferred, whereas for larger tendons or when a stronger repair is desirable, two continuous modified Kessler sutures with a 3 to 0 looped suture give better results.

Repair of Tendon Lacerations in Zones 3, 4, and 5

The principles of operative management of flexor tendon injuries in zones 3 and 4 are similar to those for injuries in zone 2. The potential for adhesion formation postoperatively in these zones is considerably lower. Intraoperatively, the digits should be completely flexed and extended to identify the lacerated tendon ends.[21]

The tendon repair starts from the deepest lacerated one to the most superficial, with a 3 to 0 looped modified Kessler four-strand technique. Epitendinous sutures in these areas are not required.[34]

Repair of Flexor Pollicis Longus

The proximal stump of the FPL tendon is frequently retracted deep to the thenar musculature, and usually can be identified through a separate incision in the carpal canal or distal forearm. The reason for the increased retraction of the FPL tendon compared with FDP tendons is that the FPL is a single tendon without the vincula restraint between tendons. Increased tension of this tendon can also lead to a higher rate of FPL rupture.[35]

Partial Tendon Lacerations

The appropriate management of partial tendon lacerations is still debated; partial lacerations can progress to late tendon rupture or entrapment. For lacerations involving more than 50% of the tendon cross-sectional area, a core suture should be considered. If a laceration involves less than 50%, the tendon can be repaired or debrided to avoid entrapment of the tendon.[36] Advanced imaging can be useful to select cases that require exploration.[37] Immediate active movement should be encouraged to avoid adhesions.

Management of Pulleys During Tendon Repair

The flexor tendons within the region of synovial sheaths are mainly nourished through synovial diffusion. Restoration of sheath integrity is believed to preserve nutrition of the tendons, provide them with a smooth gliding surface for tendons, and decrease peritendinous adhesions. Any increase in the size of the flexor tendons from injury, edema or tendon repair can impair in its proper gliding, especially in the area of compact pulley system such as in zone-2.[38]

After repair, the surgeon should move the finger and make sure that the repair site glides comfortably without getting stuck into any of the pulleys. If the gliding is not smooth, venting of the pulleys should be performed to allow free movement of the repair site. The A2 and A4 pulleys are functionally most important and biomechanical studies have shown that 25% of A2 and all of the A4 pulleys can be incised with little functional deficit.[39]

Complications

The most common complication is failure of the repair. Failure rate in most of the cases is less than 10%, happening during the first 2 weeks of the repair, as the repair site is weakest between 6 and 12 days. Such events are usually noticed as a feeling of loss in flexion strength. In these cases, exploration followed by repair of the failed tendon repair is necessary. If a failure occurs, it has to be treated within days of the event, before retraction and scarring could negatively influence a successful repair.[17]

The second common complication is tendon adhesions, resulting in digital stiffness with limited active movement and full passive movement. The first-line treatment is physiotherapy; if this fails, tenolysis surgery is indicated after 3 to 6 months. A prerequisite for successful tenolysis is that full or nearly full passive digital flexion has been achieved.[17]

Interphalangeal joint contracture can occur after flexor tendon repair. Early identification and treatment of the contracture usually results in satisfactory outcomes using passive stretching exercises and static progressive splints. Patients with contractures that limit hand function at 4 to 6 months after tendon repair can be considered for joint release.

Pulley rupture with resultant tendon bowstringing, quadriga effect, digital triggering, swan-neck digital deformity, and lumbrical-plus fingers can occur but are less common (**Table 1**).[40] Infection and skin flap necrosis are common complications of every type of hand surgery.[41]

Outcomes

The outcome after flexor tendon repair is variable, and depends on the nature of the injury, the patient's individual biological response, repair timing and method, and the patient ability to participate in a postoperative occupational activity.[42] Several scoring systems can help therapists to monitor rehabilitation progress: the Linear Measurement System, Buck-Gramcko, Strickland, American Society of Surgery of the Hand Total Active Motion system, Grossman and Grossman System II.[22]

Table 1 Description of the possible complications following pulley ruptures	
Tendon bowstringing	The tendon appears like a bowstring avoiding the full extension of finger
Quadriga effect	Flexion lag of the fingers adjacent to the injured finger from an excessive shortening of the injured tendon
Digital triggering	Sensation of "click" during finger flexion and inability to fully extend the finger
Swan neck digital deformity	Condition where the MCPJ are flexed, the PIPJ extended and the DIPJ flexed
Lumbrical-plus fingers	Paradoxical extension of the IP joint of one finger while attempting to flex all the other fingers (it is caused by FDP disruption distal to the origin of the lumbricals)

REHABILITATION PROTOCOLS AFTER SURGERY

Despite advances in suture methods and better understanding of the tendon repair biology, formation of adhesions between repaired tendon and the surrounding sheath with resultant digital stiffness remains the most common complication after flexor tendon repair.[43] Adhesions are, to some extent, part of the healing process; the challenge is to obtain a tenorrhaphy fine enough to ensure tendon gliding through the confined flexor pulley system and at the same time, strong enough to allow early mobilization. Early mobilization reduces adhesion formation and improves the quality of tendon healing.[44] To improve the strength at the tendon repair site, rehabilitation methods that produce increased in-vivo force across the repair have been investigated. Some studies advocated that tendon loading is beneficial, whereas more recent studies from the same group in the Mayo Clinic showed that motion rather than loading strengthen the tendon.[45,46]

However, there is insufficient evidence from randomized controlled trials to define the best mobilization strategy. Nevertheless, the zone of tendon injury is a key factor affecting the choice of rehabilitation program and clinical outcome.

Any flexor tendon repair follows physiological healing stages that might guide rehabilitation. In the early stage (0 to 3 weeks after repair), the inflammatory phase is at the beginning and the tensile strength of the flexor tendon repair site is weak. In the intermediate stage (4 to 6 weeks after repair), there is remodeling of the repaired tendon and mobilization or removing the splint can be started. In the late stage (at 6 to 8 weeks), muscle strengthening and activities of daily living can proceed.[35] Rehabilitation is significantly influenced by patient compliance, nature of the wound, and the repair process. Before beginning therapy, it is important for the therapist to have information from the surgeon about type of repair performed and whether other structures were injured. If a high-strength tendon repair technique was successfully performed in a compliant patient, a more aggressive early motion program can be started.

Zone I

Zone I rehabilitation is focused on achieving passive and active DIP joint motion to prevent adhesion formation between the A4 pulley and the FDP tendon.

Evans' protocol is recommended for end-to-end repair, advancement, or reinsertion into bone.

Zone II

Zone II rehabilitation protocols can be divided into:

- Early passive mobilization (EPM) (Kleinert protocol, Duran Houser protocol): for 2-strand sutures repair
- Early active mobilization (EAM) (Belfast and Sheffield, Strickland protocol, Silverskiold & May protocol): minimum 4-strand sutures repair
- Immobilization protocols

In a systematic review on flexor tendon rehabilitation,[47] patients who EPM showed a 4% rate of tendon ruptures and a 9% rate of decreased ROM. Patients who underwent EAM had a 5% risk of ruptures and 6% risk of decreased ROM but less than the first.

The aim of EPM was to avoid restrictive adhesion and promote intrinsic healing from synovial diffusion. The most used programs are the Kleinert and Duran&Hauser protocols.

The Kleinert Protocol consists of dynamic traction that leaves the digit in flexion. A rubber band directly connects the wrist to the fingernail of the

injured finger and, every hour, the patient actively extends the fingers to the limits of the splint 10 times (**Fig. 4**). The concept is that the elastic band acts as the repaired flexor tendon unit without flexor muscle contraction. Two complications can be observed using this protocol: flexion contractures at the PIP joint and loss of active DIP motion. To prevent the latter complication, the modified Kleinert program adds a palmar pulley to improve DIP flexion.[48]

The Duran and Houser protocol (**Fig. 5**) starts on the third day after surgery with the patient's passive flexion and extension of the PIP joint of the affected finger while holding the DIP and MP joints flexed. Then, the patient passively moves the DIP joint into extension and flexion with the MP and PIP joints flexed. After 4.5 weeks, active extension and passive flexion of the distal interphalangeal joint (DIP) and PIP joints begin within the constraints of the splint.[24]

Duran and colleagues[49] reported that 3 to 5 mm of tendon excursion were sufficient to prevent restrictive adhesions after repair.

EAM aims to increase the amount of tendon excursion within the sheath and improve outcomes but does not accelerate tendon healing. Most published protocols start motion at 24 to 48 h after surgery because the resistance to flexion imposed by the surrounding edematous tissues is less, but all protocols use a dorsal blocking splint and protect the tendon by limiting active flexion for the first 3 to 6 weeks (**Table 2**). EAM protocols depend on strong repair techniques and the force applied during rehabilitation must be less than the tensile strength of the repair to prevent gapping or rupture.

When children or adolescents under 10 years sustain a lacerated tendon and undergo repair, the decision whether the patient is a candidate for an early motion program should be taken with

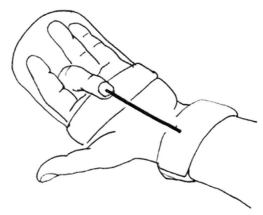

Fig. 4. Rubber band that connects the wrist to the fingernail directly.

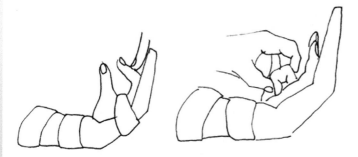

Fig. 5. Passive mobilization of the fingers.

help from the parents and treating therapist. Indeed, the early motion flexor tendon rehabilitation program requires that the child is mature enough to perform the essential functions of rehabilitation safely. The same procedure should be followed in patients with cognitive deficits, patients unable or unwilling to participate in a complex rehabilitation program, or patients who must protect other injuries (fractures for examples). If the decision is not to allow an early motion program, the patient's wrist and hand are immobilized

3 or 4 weeks in a dorsal forearm-based splint holding the wrist in 10° to 30° of flexion, the MP joints in 40° to 60° of flexion, and the IP joints initially in slight flexion and at the first appointment in full extension.[50] The splint is worn 24 h a day except for therapy visits (one to two times a week).

Zone III

Zone III rehabilitation is described by Al-Qattan.[21] Patients perform mobilization exercises daily at

Table 2
Dorsal blocking splint at the first stages

	Wrist	MCP	PIP	IP	DIP
Evan	30° to 40° flexion	30 flexion			40° to 45° flexion
Kleinert	45° flexion	10° to 20° flexion	Full extension allowed	Full extension allowed	Full extension allowed
Duran Hauser	20°flexion	50° to 60° flexion	Full extension allowed	Full extension allowed	Full extension allowed
Belfast sheffield[51]	30° to 40° flexion	80° to 90° flexion	Full extension allowed	Full extension allowed	Full extension allowed
Strickland dorsal blocking splint[52]	20° of flexion and 30° of extension allowed	50° of flexion	Full flexion and extension allowed	Full flexion and extension allowed	Full flexion and extension allowed
Strickland exercise splint[52]	Full flexion and 30° of extension allowed	50° of flexion and 60° of extension allowed	Full flexion and extension allowed	Full flexion extension allowed	Full flexion and extension allowed
Silfverskiold and May[53]	Neutral position	50° to 70° of flexion	Full extension allowed	Full extension allowed	Full extension allowed
Al Qattan[54]	Neutral position	30° of flexion	Full extension allowed	Full extension allowed	Full extension allowed
Indiana Hand Protocol[22]	20°of flexion	65° to 70° of flexion	0° of flexion, extension allowed	0° of flexion, extension allowed	0° of flexion, extension allowed
Modified Duran and Kleinert[23]	30° of flexion	50° of flexion	Full extension allowed	Full extension allowed	Full extension allowed

home and visit a hand therapist twice weekly. They can extend their fingers actively wearing a splint.

After 4 weeks, the splint is removed, and active flexion and extension is performed without resistance. Active flexion against resistance is started 6 weeks after surgery.[22]

Zone IV

Zone IV rehabilitation follows the Indiana Hand Protocol. A dorsal blocking splint is used, and composite passive flexion extension can be performed on each finger by the patient until the third week. After that, blocking exercises promote tendon gliding and minimize scar contracture.[22]

Zone V

Zone V rehabilitation provides good results in patients treated with surgical repair,modified Duran and modified Kleinert rehabilitation protocols can be used. The protocol involves passive flexion and active extension of the injured fingers of the injured hand on the second or third postoperative day for 4 weeks.[23]

Flexor Pollicis Longus

FPL rehabilitation follows the EAM protocols described for zone II injuries. An adaptation of either EAM or the Kleinert technique is used.[35]

Adjuvant Therapy

To obtain better gliding of the hand flexor tendons by reducing peritendinous adhesions without adversely affecting the healing process itself, some options have been explored. Given the adhesiogenic nature of tendon repair, drugs, and biological barriers have been studied to prevent adhesion formation.[55]

Several drugs influence the healing inflammatory phase and inhibit fibroblast proliferation suppressing pro-adhesion formation growth factors. These include hyaluronic acid, nonsteroidal anti-inflammatory drugs (Ibuprofen and Indomethacin), 5-fluorouracil, human amniotic fluid, alginate solution, collagen synthesis inhibitor (CPHI-I), enriched collagen solution, plant alkaloid halofuginone, human-derived fibrin sealant, topical β-aminopropionitrile, and transforming GFβ-1 inhibitors.[24] Biocompatible barrier between surrounding tissues and the repaired tendon may be able to further reduce the formation of adhesions without interfering with the nutrition and healing. Polytetrafluoroethene, hydroxyapatite, hyaluronic acid membrane, polyvinyl alcohol hydrogel, and bovine pericardium have been tried[56,57]

Other modalities such as ultrasound therapy and pulsed electromagnetic field have also been tried but only animal studies with controversial results are available.[57]

Future Therapies

Gene therapy in hand flexor tendon surgery has been proposed using adenoviral, adeno-associated viral (AAV), and liposome plasmid vectors able to deliver genes to tendons improving their healing. However, clinical evidence is lacking.[58]

SUMMARY

Tendon biology and anatomy are crucial to manage hand flexor tendon injuries, not only for surgical treatment but also for rehabilitation; surgeon and physical therapist have to choose zone by zone as the best way to manage and restore the normal function of hand flexor tendons.

CLINICS CARE POINTS

- In Zone I, tendon-to-bone repair can be obtained through traditional pull-out suture methods or internal suture methods. When the distal tendon stump is longer than 1 cm, primary tenorrhaphy is preferred. Evans' protocol is recommended for rehabilitation.

- In Zone II, tendon repair with double-strand or four-strand core suture placement is preferred. Early passive mobilisation (EPM), early active mobilisation (EAM) or Immobilization protocols are all available rehabilitation programs.

- In Zone III, IV and V, the principles of operative management are similar to those for injuries in zone 2. The tendon repair is obtained with a 3-0 looped modified Kessler four-strand technique. Epitendinous sutures in these areas are not required. Zone III rehabilitation is described by Al-Qattan, while Zone IV rehabilitation follows the Indiana Hand Protocol. Zone V rehabilitation provides good results in patients treated with modified Duran and modified Kleinert rehabilitation protocols.

- The most common complications of hand flexor tendon repair are failure and tendon adhesions.

FUNDING

The authors did not receive any funding.

DISCLOSURE

The authors have no potential conflicts of interest.

REFERENCES

1. Lister GD, Kleinert HE, Kutz JE, et al. Primary flexor tendon repair followed by immediate controlled mobilization. J Hand Surg Am 1977;2(6):441–51.
2. Aicale R, Tarantino D, Maffulli N. Basic science of tendons. Bio-orthopaedics: a new approach 2017. p. 249–73.
3. Aicale R, Tarantino D, Maccauro G, et al. Genetics in orthopaedic practice. J Biol Regul Homeost Agents 2019;33(2 Suppl. 1):103–17.
4. Aicale R, Tarantino D, Maffulli N. Overuse injuries in sport: a comprehensive overview. J Orthopaedic Surg Res 2018;13(1):309.
5. Elliott DH. Structure and function of mammalian tendon. Biol Rev Camb Philos Soc 1965;40: 392–421.
6. Kvist M, Jozsa L, Kannus P, et al. Morphology and histochemistry of the myotendineal junction of the rat calf muscles. histochemical, immunohistochemical and electron-microscopic study. Acta Anat (Basel) 1991;141(3):199–205.
7. Aicale R, Tarantino D, Maffulli N. Surg tendinopathies. Sports Med Arthrosc Rev 2018;26(4):200–2.
8. Benjamin M, Ralphs JR. Fibrocartilage in tendons and ligaments–an adaptation to compressive load. J Anat 1998;193(Pt 4):481–94.
9. Benjamin M, Qin S, Ralphs JR. Fibrocartilage associated with human tendons and their pulleys. J Anat 1995;187(Pt 3):625–33.
10. Evans EJ, Benjamin M, Pemberton DJ. Fibrocartilage in the attachment zones of the quadriceps tendon and patellar ligament of man. J Anat 1990; 171:155–62.
11. de Albornoz PM, Aicale R, Forriol F, et al. Cell therapies in tendon, ligament, and musculoskeletal system repair. Sports Med Arthrosc Rev 2018;26(2): 48–58.
12. Lundborg G, Myrhage R. The vascularization and structure of the human digital tendon sheath as related to flexor tendon function. an angiographic and histological study. Scand J Plast Reconstr Surg 1977;11(3):195–203.
13. Strickland JW. Development of flexor tendon surgery: twenty-five years of progress. J Hand Surg Am 2000;25(2):214–35.
14. Ochiai N, Matsui T, Miyaji N, et al. Vascular anatomy of flexor tendons. I. Vincular system and blood supply of the profundus tendon in the digital sheath. J Hand Surg Am 1979;4(4):321–30.
15. Lundborg G, Rank F. Experimental intrinsic healing of flexor tendons based upon synovial fluid nutrition. J Hand Surg Am 1978;3(1):21–31.
16. Allan CH. Flexor tendons: anatomy and surgical approaches. Hand Clin 2005;21(2):151–7.
17. Dy CJ, Hernandez-Soria A, Ma Y, et al. Complications after flexor tendon repair: a systematic review and meta-analysis. J Hand Surg 2012;37(3): 543–51.e1.
18. Leddy JP, Packer JW. Avulsion of the profundus tendon insertion in athletes. J Hand Surg Am 1977; 2(1):66–9.
19. Trumble TE, Vedder NB, Benirschke SK. Misleading fractures after profundus tendon avulsions: a report of six cases. J Hand Surg Am 1992;17(5):902–6.
20. Dy CJ, Daluiski A. Update on zone II flexor tendon injuries. J Am Acad Orthop Surg 2014;22(12):791–9.
21. Al-Qattan MM. Flexor tendon repair in zone III. J Hand Surg Eur Vol 2011;36(1):48–52.
22. Klifto CS, Bookman J, Paksima N. Postsurgical rehabilitation of flexor tendon injuries. J Hand Surg Am 2019;44(8):680–6.
23. Bircan C, El O, Akalin E, et al. Functional outcome in patients with zone V flexor tendon injuries. Arch Orthop Trauma Surg 2005;125(6):405–9.
24. Boyer MI, Strickland JW, Engles D, et al. Flexor tendon repair and rehabilitation: state of the art in 2002. Instr Course Lect 2003;52:137–61.
25. Lutsky KF, Giang EL, Matzon JL. Flexor tendon injury, repair and rehabilitation. Orthop Clin North Am 2015;46(1):67–76.
26. Komanduri M, Phillips CS, Mass DP. Tensile strength of flexor tendon repairs in a dynamic cadaver model. J Hand Surg Am 1996;21(4):605–11.
27. Gelberman RH, Boyer MI, Brodt MD, et al. The effect of gap formation at the repair site on the strength and excursion of intrasynovial flexor tendons. an experimental study on the early stages of tendon-healing in dogs. J Bone Joint Surg Am 1999;81(7): 975–82.
28. Chauhan A, Palmer BA, Merrell GA. Flexor tendon repairs: techniques, eponyms, and evidence. J Hand Surg Am 2014;39(9):1846–53.
29. McCallister WV, Ambrose HC, Katolik LI, et al. Comparison of pullout button versus suture anchor for zone I flexor tendon repair. J Hand Surg Am 2006; 31(2):246–51.
30. Silva MJ, Thomopoulos S, Kusano N, et al. Early healing of flexor tendon insertion site injuries: tunnel repair is mechanically and histologically inferior to surface repair in a canine model. J Orthop Res 2006;24(5):990–1000.
31. Buscemi MJ, Page BJ. Flexor digitorum profundus avulsions with associated distal phalanx fractures. a report of four cases and review of the literature. Am J Sports Med 1987;15(4):366–70.
32. Ruchelsman DE, Christoforou D, Wasserman B, et al. Avulsion injuries of the flexor digitorum profundus tendon. J Am Acad Orthop Surg 2011;19(3): 152–62.

33. Hage JJ. History off-hand: bunnell's no-man's land. Hand (N Y) 2019;14(4):570–4.

34. Kleinert HE, Kutz JE, Atasoy E, et al. Primary repair of flexor tendons. Orthop Clin North Am 1973;4(4): 865–76.

35. Pearce O, Brown MT, Fraser K, et al. Flexor tendon injuries: repair & rehabilitation. Injury 2021;52(8): 2053–67.

36. Bishop AT, Cooney WP, Wood MB. Treatment of partial flexor tendon lacerations: the effect of tenorrhaphy and early protected mobilization. J Trauma 1986;26(4):301–12.

37. Teefey SA, Middleton WD, Boyer MI. Sonography of the hand and wrist. Semin Ultrasound CT MR 2000; 21(3):192–204.

38. Gelberman RH, Manske PR, Akeson WH, et al. Flexor tendon repair. J Orthop Res 1986;4(1): 119–28.

39. Mitsionis G, Bastidas JA, Grewal R, et al. Feasibility of partial A2 and A4 pulley excision: effect on finger flexor tendon biomechanics. J Hand Surg Am 1999; 24(2):310–4.

40. Sandvall BK, Kuhlman-Wood K, Recor C, et al. Flexor tendon repair, rehabilitation, and reconstruction. Plast Reconstr Surg 2013;132(6):1493–503.

41. Whittaker JP, Nancarrow JD, Sterne GD. The role of antibiotic prophylaxis in clean incised hand injuries: a prospective randomized placebo controlled double blind trial. J Hand Surg Br 2005;30(2):162–7.

42. Tang JB. Clinical outcomes associated with flexor tendon repair. Hand Clin 2005;21(2):199–210.

43. Rrecaj S, Martinaj M, Murtezani A, et al. Physical therapy and splinting after flexor tendon repair in zone II. Med Arch 2014;68(2):128–31.

44. Hill C, Riaz M, Mozzam A, et al. A regional audit of hand and wrist injuries. a study of 4873 injuries. J Hand Surg Br 1998;23(2):196–200.

45. Boyer MI, Gelberman RH, Burns ME, et al. Intrasynovial flexor tendon repair. an experimental study comparing low and high levels of in vivo force during rehabilitation in canines. J Bone Joint Surg Am 2001; 83(6):891–9.

46. Boyer MI, Goldfarb CA, Gelberman RH. Recent progress in flexor tendon healing. the modulation of tendon healing with rehabilitation variables. J Hand Ther 2005;18(2):80–5 [quiz: 86].

47. Starr HM, Snoddy M, Hammond KE, et al. Flexor tendon repair rehabilitation protocols: a systematic review. J Hand Surg Am 2013;38(9):1712–7.e1-14.

48. Edinburg M, Widgerow AD, Biddulph SL. Early postoperative mobilization of flexor tendon injuries using a modification of the Kleinert technique. J Hand Surg Am 1987;12(1):34–8.

49. Duran R, Houser R, Coleman C, et al. A preliminary report in the use of controlled passive motion following flexor tendon repair in zones II and III. J Hand Surg [Am] 1976;1:79.

50. Elhassan B, Moran SL, Bravo C, et al. Factors that influence the outcome of zone I and zone II flexor tendon repairs in children. J Hand Surg Am 2006; 31(10):1661–6.

51. Kannas S, Jeardeau TA, Bishop AT. Rehabilitation following zone II flexor tendon repairs. Tech Hand Up Extrem Surg 2015;19(1):2–10.

52. Strickland JW, Glogovac SV. Digital function following flexor tendon repair in zone II: a comparison of immobilization and controlled passive motion techniques. J Hand Surg Am 1980;5(6):537–43.

53. Silfverskiöld KL, May EJ. Flexor tendon repair in zone II with a new suture technique and an early mobilization program combining passive and active flexion. J Hand Surg Am 1994;19(1):53–60.

54. Al-Qattan MM, Mirdad AT, Hafiz MO. Suture purchase length: a biomechanical study of flexor tendon repair in newborn lambs. J Hand Surg Am 2013;38(1):62–5.

55. Robbins JR, Evanko SP, Vogel KG. Mechanical loading and TGF-beta regulate proteoglycan synthesis in tendon. Arch Biochem Biophys 1997; 342(2):203–11.

56. Hanff G, Abrahamsson SO. Matrix synthesis and cell proliferation in repaired flexor tendons within e-PTFE reconstructed flexor tendon sheaths. J Hand Surg Br 1996;21(5):642–6.

57. Khanna A, Friel M, Gougoulias N, et al. Prevention of adhesions in surgery of the flexor tendons of the hand: what is the evidence? Br Med Bull 2009;90: 85–109.

58. Khanna A, Gougoulias N, Maffulli N. Modalities in prevention of flexor tendon adhesion in the hand: what have we achieved so far? Acta Orthop Belg 2009;75(4):433–44.

Pediatric Flexor Tendon Injuries

Brian W. Starr, MD[a],*, Roger Cornwall, MD[a]

KEYWORDS

- Pediatric flexor tendon • Repair • Reconstruction • Rehabilitation • Zone 2

KEY POINTS

- Smaller anatomy and the dynamics of behavioral development add complexity to pediatric flexor tendon diagnosis, repair, and rehabilitation.
- Primary, multi-strand repair should be performed whenever possible, regardless of age or zone of injury.
- Multi-strand repairs reduce the risk of flexor tendon rupture at the expense of repair-site bulkiness. Venting of A2 and A4 pulleys as necessary can be safely performed.
- Pediatric patients are generally less at risk of postoperative stiffness than adults, and young patients can be cast safely for up to 4 weeks postoperatively.

INTRODUCTION

Compared with flexor tendon injuries in the adult population, pediatric injuries are a rare entity, with a reported incidence of 3.6 injuries per 100,000 patients per year.[1] The incidence in adults is nearly 10 times greater, with an incidence of 33.2 injuries per 100,000 patients per year.[2] The majority of injuries occur in zone II, with a peak incidence in children occurring at approximately 3 years of age.[3] Sharp laceration from glass is the leading mechanism of injury; knife injuries are more common in adolescents, with a notable uptick in incidence during the pumpkin-carving season in the fall.[4,5]

The diagnosis and management of pediatric flexor tendon injuries present unique challenges to the hand surgeon. Prompt diagnosis can be complicated by the dynamics of behavioral development. Examiners should be suspicious of an injury and carefully observe how the child interacts with parents, providers, and their environment. An otherwise innocuous-appearing puncture or laceration in a young child may be accompanied by a flexor tendon or nerve injury. For these reasons, flexor tendon lacerations in young children are frequently diagnosed late—sometimes weeks or months after the inciting injury. In a recent retrospective review of patients with zone I or II flexor tendon injuries, Piper and colleagues[6] found an average interval of 21 weeks between the date of injury and surgical treatment. In addition to challenges in diagnosis, diminutive tendon caliber in small children can complicate surgical repair. In patients under 2 years of age, the flexor digitorum profundus (FDP) tendon measures just 2 to 3 mm wide by 0.5 to 1 mm thick.[5] Four- and six-strand repair techniques are supported by recent literature, though the surgeon must remain diligent to ensure gliding of a bulky repair in a narrow tendon sheath.[7] Beyond the operating room, postoperative management must be tailored to accommodate nuances specific to patient age and behavioral development. A technically sound and biomechanically strong repair may better tolerate overzealous patient participation. However, a fluid, patient-specific approach to every stage of management is critical for the successful treatment of pediatric flexor tendon injuries.

[a] Division of Orthopedic Surgery, Cincinnati Children's Hospital Medical Center, 3333 Burnet Avenue, Cincinnati, OH 45229, USA
* Corresponding author.
E-mail address: brian.starr@cchmc.org

Hand Clin 39 (2023) 227–233
https://doi.org/10.1016/j.hcl.2022.08.022

ZONE I INJURIES

As described by Moiemen and Elliot, zone I can be divided into three subzones. Zone Ia is located at the FDP insertion, where traditional core suture repair is not possible; Zone Ib is located between the distal edge of the A4 pulley and the proximal extent of zone Ia; and zone 1c spans the distance from the distal edge of the A4 pulley to the FDS insertion (distal zone 2) (**Fig. 1**).[8] Traditional approaches for the treatment of distal injuries occurring in zone Ia (ie, jersey finger) are well-described in the adult literature and include an array of bone tunnel, suture anchor, or pullout options. The classic Bunnell pullout technique, with externalized suture and button sewn over the nail plate, carries the risk of infection and nail deformity.[9] However, more recent techniques aimed at internalizing the suture are also susceptible to complications. In a biomechanical study comparing suture techniques, Chu and colleagues[10] found no statistically significant difference in ultimate load or work-to-failure between dorsally internalized suture and volar anchor techniques. However, in a separate study, Geary and colleagues[11] noted complications in five of eight patients who underwent FDP repair with internalization of the repair knot over the dorsal distal phalanx. Complications in this small series included osteomyelitis, chronic granuloma, and nail deformity. Kapickis and colleagues[12] proposed a modification of this technique in which the internalized suture is tunneled through the distal phalanx in a volar-to-dorsal fashion before being passed back dorsal-to-volar, thus allowing the knot to sit volarly, at the FDP reattachment site. This technique theoretically avoids complications such as granuloma and nail deformity resulting from dorsal knot irritation. With any of the aforementioned techniques, suture anchor or transosseous suture placement must be positioned with care. Especially in pediatric patients, avoiding iatrogenic injury to the physis or germinal matrix depends on a narrow target window. Fluoroscopy must be used to confirm proper positioning before drilling transosseous tunnels or placing suture anchors. For proximal zone I injuries occurring in zone Ib or Ic, core suture repair with or without an epitendinous suture is often possible (**Fig. 2**).

Pediatric literature specific to zone I flexor tendon injuries is relatively sparse. A 2012 review by Al-Qattan found just 55 reported cases of pediatric zone I flexor tendon lacerations. In describing his technique for treating zone I lacerations with his hallmark six-strand, triple figure-of-eight suture technique, Al-Qattan reported impressive outcomes in 22 patients ages 5 to 10 years. The six-strand

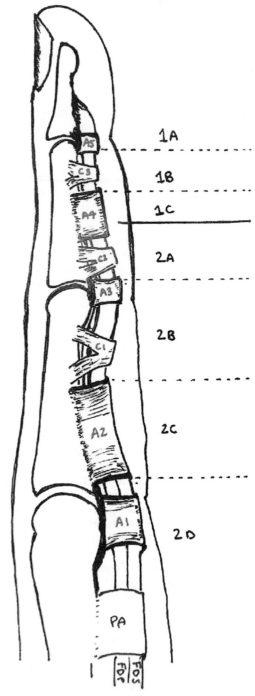

Fig. 1. Flexor tendon sheath anatomy; zone I subdivisions as described by Moiemen and Elliot[8]; zone II subdivision as described by Tang.[30] (Courtesy of Brian Starr, MD, Ann Arbor, MI.)

technique, performed with 4 to 0 polypropylene core sutures, facilitated early active motion protocols with no ruptures. In more proximal zone I injuries (Ib and Ic), repair was augmented with a 5 to

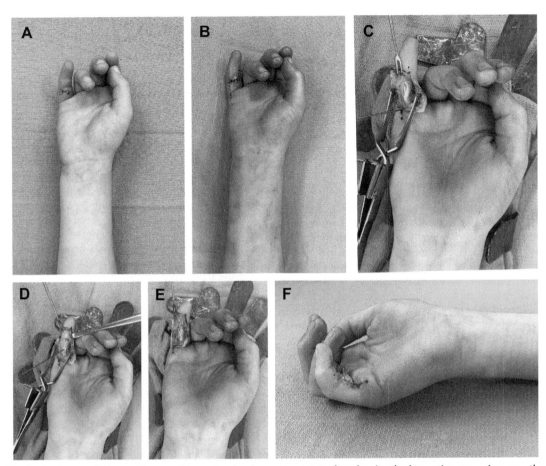

Fig. 2. An 8-year-old boy with zone I flexor tendon laceration. Note that despite the laceration occurring over the skin of P1, the sharp laceration occurred with a clenched fist, and so the tendon injury occurred in zone 1c. (*A*) Preoperative resting posture. (*B*) Preoperative mid-axial incisions marked. (*C*) Proximal stump of FDP tendon retrieved and temporarily secured with a Keith needle. Partial venting of A2 pulley. (*D*) Approximation of proximal and distal FDP ends. Preserved A4 pulley. (*E*) Four-strand repair of FDP tendon with 4-0 Ethibond suture. (*F*) Resting posture, post-repair. (Courtesy of Kevin C. Chung MD, MS.)

0 polypropylene epitendinous suture. In distal (Ia) injuries without sufficient distal tendon, the volar plate was incorporated into the distal purchase. The author notes that this technique is "very bulky" and that pulley venting is mandatory. In follow-up, all patients were reported to have "excellent" outcomes according to the Strickland and Glogovac criteria. Outcomes specific to DIP joint motion, as assessed by the Moiemen-Elliot criteria, were tempered slightly, with 64% of patients meeting the threshold for "good" or "excellent" results, whereas 36% of patients showed "fair" outcomes.[13]

SENIOR AUTHOR'S PREFERRED TECHNIQUE: ZONE I

With distal injuries in zone Ia, our preferred technique depends on the size of the distal phalanx and the presence of an open physis. In skeletally mature patients, suture anchors can be used. However, in younger patients, the presence of a physis and the very shallow dorsal-volar diameter of the distal phalanx distal to the physis conspire to preclude suture anchor placement, so in these patients, our preferred strategy is to repair the tendon to the distal phalanx with a pullout 2-0 modified Kessler nonabsorbable monofilament suture over a button dorsal to the nail plate. Fluoroscopy is used to prevent injury to the physis while a straight Keith needle is driven under power through the distal phalanx and out through the sterile matrix and nail plate, distal to the lunula. Both arms of the pullout suture are passed through this one hole before being split through the two holes of the button to tie the knot over the button. This single hole minimizes the potential nail deformity and allows optimal placement of the FDP footprint in the small area distal to the physis.

The closed rupture mechanisms that produce zone Ia injuries typically occur in patients old enough to tolerate the presence of the button over the nail, even when visible during early motion therapy protocols. The suture is cut and removed at 6 weeks postoperatively, which is again tolerated well in pediatric patients. In proximal zone I injuries (zone Ib/Ic), we routinely perform a multi-strand four- or six-strand repair and vent the A4 pulley, as indicated.

ZONE II INJURIES

As with proximal zone I injuries, multi-strand core suture repair has become the standard for most zone II flexor tendon lacerations. In a randomized controlled study comparing outcomes of two-strand versus four-strand repair techniques in pediatric patients, Navali and Rouhani reported a higher rate of rupture in patients who underwent two-strand repairs.[7] Nietosvaara and colleagues[1] reviewed outcomes of 45 pediatric flexor tendon repairs and noted a similar range of motion between two-strand and four-strand repair groups at 38 months postoperatively. Complications were notable; however, for three cases of tendon rupture—all occurring in the two-strand repair group. Owing to the diminutive tendon caliber of young children, two-strand repairs are more prevalent in children under 2 years of age. Irrespective of age, Al-Qattan advocates for a six-strand, three-figure-of-eight, method.[5,14,15] Proposed benefits of this specific technique include simplicity, reduced tendon handling, and usefulness for repairs of flat tendons because it is a full-thickness grasp, as opposed to a core suture. As expected, this technique creates a strong—but bulky—construct. For this reason, Al-Qattan advocates for FDP-only repair and proximal venting of as needed. For children under 6 years of age, 5-0 or 6-0 polypropylene core sutures are used, with a 6-0 or 7-0 epitendinous suture; patients 6 years or older are more suitable for 4-0 core and 5-0 or 6-0 epitendinous sutures.[5]

The impact of pulley venting has been studied with rigor in adult patients, with complete A4 and partial A2 venting becoming accepted practice (**Fig. 3**).[16,17] Little evidence exists regarding pulley management specific to pediatric patients. However, it is well documented that the pediatric flexor tendon sheath is narrow and susceptible to anatomic anomalies and inflammation that contribute to incomplete tendon excursion and triggering.[18] When using a bulky six-strand technique in even the smallest patients, Al-Qattan performs "liberal venting" of the flexor sheath. Though he notes "variable deficits" in total active flexion of

the distal interphalangeal joint, consistent with some degree of bowstringing, this remains preferable to poor tendon excursion due to catching at the repair site.[5]

SENIOR AUTHORS PREFERRED TECHNIQUE: ZONE II

For even the youngest patients we strive to achieve a four-strand repair using a combination of modified Kessler and horizontal mattress sutures with knots internal to the repair site if possible. The size of the suture depends on the age and size of the patient, ranging typically from 4-0 to 2-0 braided nonabsorbable sutures. Regarding purchase length, we agree with previous authors with respect to core suture tendon purchase, and aim for a purchase length of 1.5 to 2.0 times the tendon width.[5,7] A running, locking, 6-0 monofilament nonabsorbable epitendinous suture is used when the tendon size permits. Given the small size of the pediatric flexor sheath relative to the repair bulk, we routinely perform FDP-only repairs, even excising the FDS stumps, when both tendons are lacerated. Similarly, as many pediatric lacerations occur with a closed grasp, rendering the laceration and thus tenorrhaphy directly beneath the A4 pulley, we often release the A4 pulley to enable tendon excursion.

ZONE III–V INJURIES

Proximal to zone II, the absence of the constrictive flexor sheath simplifies tendon repair and postoperative rehabilitation. Repairs in zones III–V are less susceptible to complications, including rupture and adhesion formation requiring tenolysis.[19–21] Although dedicated literature regarding zones III–V, in either pediatric or adult populations, is limited, core flexor tendon principles still apply. Acute repair with a multistrand technique should be performed whenever possible. Concomitant tendon, nerve, or vascular injuries are common.[21] During the initial assessment, diligent observation is vital, to avoid missing a potential neurovascular injury.

TENDON RECONSTRUCTION

Though early primary flexor tendon repair should be performed whenever possible, it is not uncommon for young children to present in delayed fashion. With late diagnosis, single-stage grafting or two-stage reconstructive procedures may be required. Delayed repair or reconstruction is also a risk factor for digital growth restriction.[22] Historically, pediatric patients who required staged reconstruction were thought to have higher rates

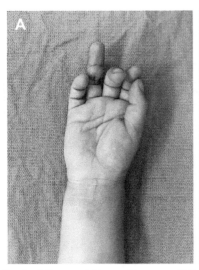
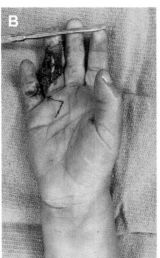
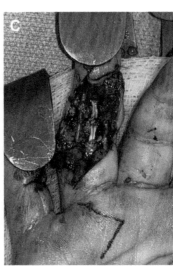

Fig. 3. A 2-year-old boy with a zone II flexor tendon laceration and concomitant transection of radial and ulnar digital nerves. A six-strand repair of the FDP tendon was completed using a modified Kessler suture in combination with two figure-of-eight sutures. The primary repair was completed with 5-0 polypropylene suture and augmented with a 6-0 polypropylene running epitendinous suture. Radial and ulnar digital nerves were repaired using a 10-0 nylon suture under the operating microscope. (*A*) Preoperative resting posture. (*B*) Exposure and repair of FDP tendon. Note partial A2 venting proximally. (*C*) Radial and ulnar digital nerves repaired with a10-0 nylon suture.

of failures and complications than adults. Amadio reported a series of 12 children (mean age 8.4 years) treated with staged flexor tendon reconstruction, with just 23% of patients achieving "good" results after staged flexor tendon reconstruction.[23] Recent literature has been more encouraging. In a review of seven children (mean age 11 years) treated with single-stage zone I or zone II flexor tendon reconstruction, Yamazaki reported good or excellent results in six patients (86%).[24] In a recent retrospective review of patients under 6 years presenting with zone I or zone II flexor tendon injuries, Piper and colleagues found that, on average, 18 weeks had passed from the time of injury for digits amenable to single-stage reconstruction. This time interval ballooned to 24 weeks in patients who required two-stage reconstruction. The authors reported a higher proportion of single-stage reconstructions achieving "good" or "excellent" results (71%) compared with the two-stage reconstruction group (40%). Piper and colleagues[6] assert that staged flexor tendon reconstruction is a viable option in patients under 6 years of age, despite diminished total active motion and Pediatric Outcomes Data Collection Instrument (PODCI) scores at mean 8 years follow-up.

Specific techniques of pediatric flexor tendon reconstruction do not differ substantially from those in adults, with the exception of the size of the flexor sheath precluding the use of standard

tendon prostheses in the first stage of a two-stage reconstruction in the smallest patients. In these patients, silicone vessel loops can be used instead.

POSTOPERATIVE MANAGEMENT AND REHABILITATION

Although adult flexor tendon rehabilitation has notably shifted toward early active range of motion protocols, pediatric protocols are frequently more restrictive because of chronologic age and behavioral risk factors. Above-elbow cast immobilization for up to 4 weeks postoperatively is the treatment of choice for young children. When applying the cast, the palm should be padded with soft, compressible dressing material that effectively prevents isometric tendon loading against the internal surface of the hard cast material.

In a recent review of 28 patients (mean age 11.4 years) with 34 injured digits, Lin and Samora reported 86% "good" or "excellent" results for zone I and II injuries treated with 4 weeks of strict immobilization followed by a modified Duran protocol.[25] Cooper and colleagues[26] reported 82% "good" or "excellent" results (and one rupture) in 63 digits treated with a modified early active mobilization protocol. For patients under 5 years of age, the authors used a boxing glove type of immobilization, with the digits rolled into flexion in the palm, for the first 4 weeks. Patients 5 years and older were treated with a variation of a dorsal blocking splint with a volar protective cage to prevent hand use. The sole rupture in this series occurred in an eight-year-old child.

Post-repair flexor tendon rupture rates range from 3% to 15%.[1,27,28] Risk factors associated with rupture include male sex, two-strand repair, and below-elbow splinting.[1,7] Immobilization is better tolerated in children than in adults. However, cast immobilization should not be used for more than 4 weeks, as longer immobilization increases the risk of stiffness without decreasing the risk of rupture.[27] Stiffness requiring tenolysis is rare in pediatric patients. Children frequently show the ability to resolve stiffness through ongoing therapy, play, and daily activities. Flexor tenolysis may be considered in patients over the age of 10 years who present with a significant discrepancy between active and passive range of motion (passive > active).[29]

SUMMARY

The management of pediatric flexor tendon injuries is a challenging endeavor for even experienced hand surgeons. Delayed presentation, smaller anatomy, and lack of cooperation often complicate treatment. In most cases, a four- or six-strand primary repair should be performed in the acute setting. Tendon gliding should be confirmed in the operating room, following repair, and proximal pulleys vented as needed. Most patients achieve "good" or "excellent" outcomes in cases of primary repair and primary grafting. Recovery is less predictable and can be suboptimal in patients who require staged reconstruction.

CLINICS CARE POINTS

- Pediatric flexor tendon repair should be performed using a multi-strand four- or six-strand technique in most patients, regardless of age or zone of injury.

- Zone Ia injuries are not amenable to direct repair and require incorporating the distal palmar plate into the repair versus tendon re-insertion method. Care should be taken to avoid iatrogenic injury to the physis or the germinal matrix with transosseous techniques.

- Bulky, multistrand repairs in zone II necessitate pulley venting. Complete A4 and partial A2 venting is well-tolerated.

- In cases of significantly delayed presentation, single-stage reconstruction with palmaris or plantaris tendon interposition tendon grafting can achieve excellent results.

- Pediatric patients are better-equipped to resolve postoperative stiffness and rarely require tenolysis procedures. Postoperative casting for up to 4 weeks is well-tolerated in young patients.

DISCLOSURES

The authors have received no funding for this article and have no relevant disclosures to report.

REFERENCES

1. Nietosvaara Y, Lindfors NC, Palmu S, et al. Flexor tendon injuries in pediatric patients. J Hand Surg Am 2007;32(10):1549–57.

2. de Jong JP, Nguyen JT, Sonnema AJ, et al. The incidence of acute traumatic tendon injuries in the hand and wrist: A 10-year population-based study. Clin Orthop Surg 2014;6(2):196–202.

3. Berndtsson L, Ejeskär A. Zone II flexor tendon repair in children. A retrospective long term study. Scand J Plast Reconstr Surg Hand Surg 1995;29(1):59–64.

4. Sikora S, Lai M, Arneja JS. Pediatric flexor tendon injuries: A 10-year outcome analysis. Can J Plast Surg 2013;21(3):181–5. cjps21181 [pii].

5. Al-Qattan MM. Flexor tendon injuries in the child. J Hand Surg Eur 2014;39(1):46–53.

6. Piper SL, Wheeler LC, Mills JK, et al. Outcomes after primary repair and staged reconstruction of zone I and II flexor tendon injuries in children. J Pediatr Orthop 2019;39(5):263.

7. Navali AM, Rouhani A. Zone 2 flexor tendon repair in young children: A comparative study of four-strand versus two-strand repair. J Hand Surg Eur 2008; 33(4):424–9.

8. Moiemen NS, Elliot D. Primary flexor tendon repair in zone 1. J Hand Surg Br 2000;25(1):78–84. S0266-7681(99)90319-4 [pii].

9. Kang N, Marsh D, Dewar D. The morbidity of the button-over-nail technique for zone 1 flexor tendon repairs. should we still be using this technique? J Hand Surg Eur 2008;33(5):566–70.

10. Chu JY, Chen T, Awad HA, et al. Comparison of an all-inside suture technique with traditional pull-out suture and suture anchor repair techniques for flexor digitorum profundus attachment to bone. J Hand Surg Am 2013;38(6):1084–90. S0363-5023(13) 00241-4 [pii].

11. Geary MB, Li KK, Chadderdon RC, et al. Complications following transosseous repair of zone I flexor tendon injuries. J Hand Surg Am 2020;45(12): 1183.e1–7. S0363-5023(20)30339-7 [pii].

12. Kapickis M. New "loop" suture for FDP zone I injuries. Tech Hand Up Extrem Surg 2009;13(3): 141–4.

13. Al-Qattan MM. Zone I flexor profundus tendon repair in children 5-10 years of age using 3 "figure of eight" sutures followed by immediate active mobilization. Ann Plast Surg 2012;68(1):29–32.

14. Al-Qattan MM. A six-strand technique for zone II flexor-tendon repair in children younger than 2 years of age. Injury 2011;42(11):1262–5.

15. Al-Qattan MM. Finger zone II flexor tendon repair in children (5-10 years of age) using three 'figure of eight' sutures followed by immediate active mobilization. J Hand Surg Eur 2011;36(4):291–6.

16. Kwai Ben I, Elliot D. Venting" or partial lateral release of the A2 and A4 pulleys after repair of zone 2 flexor tendon injuries. J Hand Surg Br 1998;23(5):649–54.

17. Tang JB. Release of the A4 pulley to facilitate zone II flexor tendon repair. J Hand Surg Am 2014;39(11): 2300–7. S0363-5023(14)01168-X [pii].

18. Bauer AS, Bae DS. Pediatric trigger digits. J Hand Surg Am 2015;40(11):2304–9. quiz: 2309.

19. Yii NW, Urban M, Elliot D. A prospective study of flexor tendon repair in zone 5. J Hand Surg Br 1998;23(5):642–8.

20. Al-Qattan MM. Flexor tendon repair in zone III. J Hand Surg Eur 2011;36(1):48–52.

21. Athwal GS, Wolfe SW. Treatment of acute flexor tendon injury: Zones III-V. Hand Clin 2005;21(2): 181–6.

22. Cunningham MW, Yousif NJ, Matloub HS, et al. Retardation of finger growth after injury to the flexor tendons. J Hand Surg Am 1985;10(1):115–7.

23. Amadio PC. Staged flexor tendon reconstruction in children. Ann Chir Main Memb Super 1992;11(3): 194–9.

24. Yamazaki H, Kato H, Uchiyama S, et al. Long term results of early active extension and passive flexion mobilization following one-stage tendon grafting for neglected injuries of the flexor digitorum profundus in children. J Hand Surg Eur 2011;36(4):303–7.

25. Lin JS, Balch Samora J. Functional outcomes of a modified duran postoperative rehabilitation protocol after primary repairs of pediatric hand flexor tendon injuries. J Pediatr Orthop. B. 2021. https://doi.org/10.1097/BPB.0000000000000944.

26. Cooper L, Khor W, Burr N, et al. Flexor tendon repairs in children: Outcomes from a specialist tertiary centre. J Plast Reconstr Aesthet Surg 2015;68(5): 717–23. S1748-6815(14)00726-8 [pii].

27. Fitoussi F, Lebellec Y, Frajman JM, et al. Zone I and II flexor tendon laceration in children. Rev Chir Orthop Reparatrice Appar Mot 1999;85(7):684–8.

28. Elhassan B, Moran SL, Bravo C, et al. Factors that influence the outcome of zone I and zone II flexor tendon repairs in children. J Hand Surg Am 2006; 31(10):1661–6.

29. Birnie RH, Idler RS. Flexor tenolysis in children. J Hand Surg Am 1995;20(2):254–7.

30. Tang JB. Flexor tendon repair in zone 2C. J Hand Surg Br 1994;19(1):72–5.

Zone 1 Flexor Tendon Repairs
Laceration and Avulsion Injuries

Saral J. Patel, MBBS, MS[a], Andrew J. Miller, MD[a,b], A. Lee Osterman, MD[a,b],
Rowena McBeath, MD, PhD[a,b,*]

KEYWORDS

• Zone 1 • Avulsion • Enthesis • Distal phalanx

KEY POINTS

• Zone 1 flexor tendon injuries encompass laceration as well as avulsion mechanisms.
• Factors important to zone 1 flexor tendon healing include strong tendon repair techniques as well as tendon-bone fixation methods.
• Early identification and treatment of zone 1 injuries enable repair versus reconstruction or fusion.
• Outcomes after zone 1 flexor tendon repair include persistent distal interphalangeal joint flexion contracture and stiffness.

 Video content accompanies this article at http://www.hand.theclinics.com.

INTRODUCTION

Tendon injuries in the hand occur at a rate of 33.2 per 100000 person-years, with 4% of them being zone 1 flexor tendon injuries.[1] In contrast to other zones, flexor tendon injuries in zone 1 include avulsion as well as laceration mechanisms. Flexor tendon avulsions constitute closed flexor tendon injuries involving the flexor digitorum profundus (FDP) tendon distal to the insertion of flexor digitorum superficialis (FDS) tendon. The mechanism of injury is forced extension of a flexed digit, which results in an injury to the weakest point of FDP tendon at its insertion on the base of distal phalanx.[2] The injury occurs most commonly in the ring finger, as the insertion of FDP in ring finger is weaker than the middle finger.[3] Also, the ring finger is the most prominent digit during grip, making it more prone to injury.[4]

DIAGNOSIS

In flexor tendon lacerations, patients present with history of a sharp penetrating wound, sign of skin laceration, and loss of active flexion at the distal interphalangeal (DIP) joint. In flexor tendon avulsions, patients present with pain and tenderness on the volar aspect of the injured finger with no visible wound. In both injury mechanisms, on examination of the DIP joint while stabilizing the PIP joint in full extension, active flexion at DIP joint is absent. In injuries to the flexor pollicis longus (FPL) tendon of the thumb, active flexion at the IP joint is absent.

Standard anteroposterior and lateral radiographs are obtained to rule out fractures or bony avulsions. In acute cases, ultrasound or MRI may be used to assess tendon anatomy, especially if there is no bony injury on radiographs. In chronic cases, ultrasound is used to evaluate tendon retraction and help guide further treatment.

ANATOMY

Kleinert and colleagues[5] and Verdan and colleagues[6] classified flexor tendon injuries into zones as outlined in **Fig. 1**. In the fingers, zone 1

a Philadelphia Hand to Shoulder Center, Philadelphia, PA, USA; b Department of Orthopaedic Surgery, Thomas Jefferson University, Philadelphia, PA, USA
* Corresponding author. 1203 Langhorne Newtown Road, Suite 334, Langhorne, PA 19047.
E-mail address: rmcbeath@handcenters.com

Hand Clin 39 (2023) 235–250
https://doi.org/10.1016/j.hcl.2023.01.001
0749-0712/23/© 2023 Published by Elsevier Inc.

injuries affect the FDP tendon distal to the FDS insertion and, in the thumb, zone 1 injuries affect the FPL tendon distal to the oblique pulley. The FDS tendon enters each digit through the A1 pulley and divides into 2 tendon slips. The radial and ulnar slips move laterally and dorsally around the FDP tendon, rejoin at Camper's chiasm, and insert on the volar aspect of the middle phalanx as 2 separate slips (**Fig. 2**). The flexor tendons pass through a series of pulley mechanisms, which consist of thick annular pulleys and flexible cruci-

the A4 pulley), zone 1c (immediately beneath or just proximal to the A4 pulley), and zone 1p (pull-off injuries).[9]

Preoperative Planning

The goal of surgery is to achieve strong tendon repair and/or bony fixation able to withstand early motion rehabilitation. The choice of the surgical option depends on the mechanism of injury, chronicity of the injury, the size of the bone fragment, the type of avulsion, and associated injures.[10]

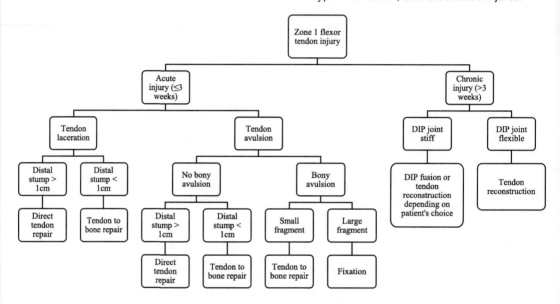

form pulleys. The flexor tendons receive blood supply from the vincular systems, osseous bony insertion, reflected vessels from the tendon sheath, and longitudinal vessels from the palm.[7,8] The vincular system can prevent retraction of the proximal tendon if undisrupted in the injury.

Zone 1 flexor tendon injuries differ from all other zones in that zone 1 includes the tendon-bone insertion, also known as the enthesis. Although most flexor tendon injuries occur from sharp lacerations and occasional puncture mechanisms, zone 1 injuries also include tendon avulsion from its insertion. The mechanism of zone 1 flexor tendon avulsion includes forced extension of a flexed digit and is commonly known as a "jersey finger."[2] Leddy and Packer[2] have classified zone 1 avulsion injuries into 5 different types as outlined in **Table 1**.

In their analysis of zone 1 injuries, Moiemen and Elliott[9] divided zone 1 flexor tendon injuries into 3 subzones: zone 1a (where the tendon is so close to its bony insertion as to inhibit suture fixation), zone 1b (between zone 1a and the distal edge of

Preparation and Patient Position

The surgery is performed in supine position with the affected limb on the hand table. Wide awake anesthesia without tourniquet is preferred, as it allows to assess gapping and gliding of the tendon repair.[11] Generally, sedation is not used in wide awake procedures unless it is used in a hybrid fashion and the patient is later woken from sedation to test the repair and tendon gliding. For chronic injuries with concern of significant tendon retraction and in cases where early active motion will not be considered, general anesthesia may be considered.

Procedural Approach

The choice of the surgical approach depends on the injury mechanism and wound pattern in case of lacerations. The options are as follows:

- Midaxial approach: preserves the normal tissue over the tendon sheath and reduces

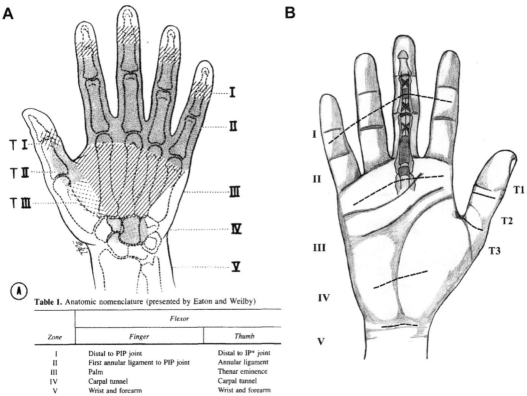

Table I. Anatomic nomenclature (presented by Eaton and Weilby)

Zone	Flexor	
	Finger	Thumb
I	Distal to PIP joint	Distal to IP* joint
II	First annular ligament to PIP joint	Annular ligament
III	Palm	Thenar eminence
IV	Carpal tunnel	Carpal tunnel
V	Wrist and forearm	Wrist and forearm

Fig. 1. Pictorial representation of flexor tendon zones of injury as originally described by Kleinert and Verdan. (*A*) Zones of flexor tendon injury as described by location. (*B*) Zones of flexor tendon injury of the finger correlating to pulley location. *Inter-Phalangeal. (*Adapted from* Ochiai N, Matsui T, Miyaji M, Merklin RJ, and Hunter JM. Vascular anatomy of flexor tendons. I. Vincular system and blood supply of the profundus tendon in the digital sheath. Journal of Hand Surgery 1979. (4) 4: 321-330; and Azar CA, Culver JE, Fleegler EJ. Blood supply of the flexor pollicis longus tendon. J Hand Surg Am. 1983 Jul;8(4):471-5; with permission.)

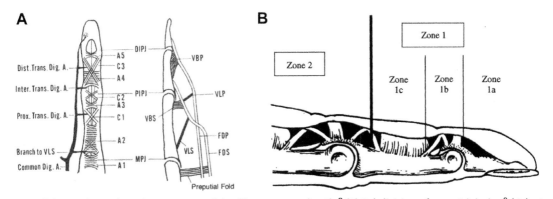

Fig. 2. (*A*) Vascular and tendon anatomy of the fibro-osseous sheath.[8] (*B*) Subdivision of zone 1 injuries.[9] (*Adapted from* Moiemen NS and Elliot D. Primary flexor tendon repair in zone 1. Journal of Hand Surgery (British and European Volume) 2000 25B: 1: 78-84; and Azar CA, Culver JE, Fleegler EJ. Blood supply of the flexor pollicis longus tendon. J Hand Surg Am. 1983 Jul;8(4):471-5; with permission.)

Table 1
Different types of zone 1 avulsion injuries

Type	Location of FDP Stump	Status of Vincula	Bony Injuries
I	FDP in palm	Vincula system disrupted	None
II	FDP at level of A3	Vincula longus profundus intact	Small avulsion fracture may or may not be present
III	FDP at level of A4	Both vincula intact	Large avulsion fracture
IV	FDP in palm	Vincula system disrupted	Large bony avulsion with detachment of FDP from the bony fragment
V	FDP at level of A4	—	Large avulsion fracture along with distal phalanx fracture

wound tension during early postoperative therapy.

- Bruner approach: it is the most widely used approach that provides wide exposure to the injured tendon.
- Volar midline longitudinal approach: the approach starts 0.5 to 1 cm distal to the volar DIP joint flexion crease and can be extended proximally as a Bruner incision. The approach provides direct visualization of the injured tendon.

A separate incision can be used to identify the proximal end of the tendon if it is retracted in the palm. Preservation of A1 is important if there is concern for disrupted flexor pulleys distally. The retracted tendon is passed through the pulley system and brought to the injury site using a small feeding tube or tendon passer, with the wrist in flexion. A milking manuever can often aid in feeding the proximal tendon distally if there is retraction. A 22-gauge needle can be placed through the tendon and A4 pulley to prevent the retraction of the tendon. In case of a large segmental defect or chronically retracted tendon, gentle pull and longitudinal traction for several minutes can provide sufficient excursion for a primary repair. However, in case of a persistent large defect, a tendon graft may be necessary.

Tendon-to-tendon repair

It is performed when the distal stump is more than 1 cm long.

Different types of tendon-to-tendon repairs include the following:

- Two-strand suture methods (Kessler, modified Kessler, or Tajima techniques)
- Four-strand suture methods (Winters-Gelberman)
- Six-strand suture methods (Tsuge repair, Tajima-Strickland, M-Tang repair)

It is essential to perform epitendinous repair to imbricate the repair site to facilitate improved gliding, to increase the strength of repair site by approximately 10% to 50%, and to decrease adhesions of the repaired tendons.[12]

The strength of the repair can be improved by

- Suture type: braided suture has a greater strength
- Suture caliber: 3-0 or 4-0 sutures
- Number of core suture strands crossing the repair site
- "Locking" core suture

If the repaired tendon is unable to pass through the A4 pulley, the pulley should be step-cut or divided. The A4 pulley should be repaired or reconstructed with local tissue or free tendon graft if the A3 pulley is not intact and bowstringing is appreciated.

Tendon-to-bone repair

It is performed when the distal stump is less than 1 cm long. The techniques of tendon-to-bone repairs can be classified into 3 categories.

- External fixation techniques: in these techniques, the sutures placed in the tendon are tied externally over a button/K-wire—for example,. Bunnell technique, Mantero technique, Grant technique, and Zhang technique.[13] Complications seen with these methods are high infection rate, abnormal nail growth, and gapping of the repair.
- Internal fixation techniques: in these techniques, the sutures are tied after passing them through transosseous drill holes (eg, Tripathi, Yeo, Sood, Kapickis method), or using bone anchors.[13] Placing bone anchors in a 45 retrograde fashion decreases gapping and prevents penetration of the dorsal cortex. Two microanchors with 4-strand repairs

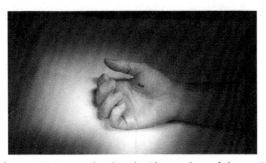

Fig. 3. Clinical photograph of zone 1 injury to the thumb. Observe loss of the resting flexed position of the IPJ.

require higher force to failure as compared with 2-strand pullout techniques.[14]

- Mixed techniques: Lee and colleagues described a new technique that uses both a pullout suture and bone anchors.[15] Bone anchors fix the tendon to the bone, and the pullout sutures augment the anchor repair.

Bone-to-bone repair

Large avulsions can be fixed by using K-wires or a 1.3- or 1.5-mm screw placed volar to dorsal. Care must be taken to avoid dorsal penetration.

Small avulsions are treated using the bone-to-tendon repair techniques.

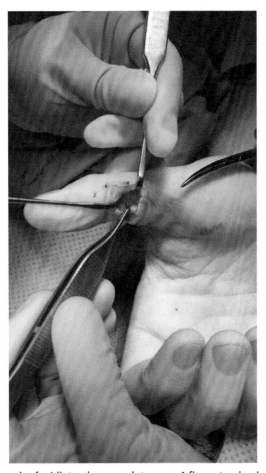

Fig. 4. Intraoperative photograph of midlateral approach to zone 1 flexor tendon laceration. The proximal end is easily identified.

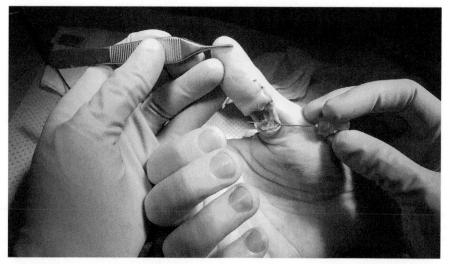

Fig. 5. Intraoperative photograph of zone 1 flexor tendon laceration, proximal end held by 25-gauge hypodermic needle. Note presence of vinculae at the dorsal aspect, preventing retraction of the tendon.

Joint fusion/salvage
In cases where the joint is stiff or the patient does not need motion, DIP fusions, particularly in chronic cases, may be considered.

Recovery and Rehabilitation Management

- A splint is applied with the wrist flexed at 20 to 30 degrees, the MCP joints flexed at 50 to 70 degrees, and the interphalangeal (IP) joints fully extended. Depending on injury mechanism, early active motion is encouraged. For avulsion injures including a bone component, passive blocking exercises can be initiated within the first week postoperatively.
- After 4 weeks, the splint is gradually extended to provide more tension at the suture site, and the patient can start active flexion exercises.

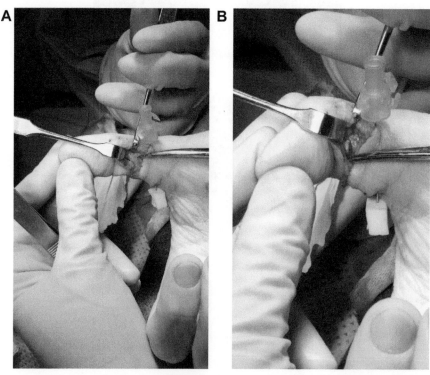

Fig. 6. Intraoperative photograph of zone 1 flexor tendon laceration: (*A*) intact oblique pulley and (*B*) distal tendon end.

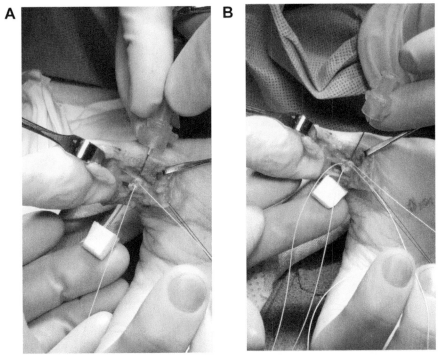

Fig. 7. Intraoperative photograph of zone 1 flexor tendon repair: (*A*) initial and (*B*) final throws of 4-0 cruciate repair using 3-0 Ethibond.

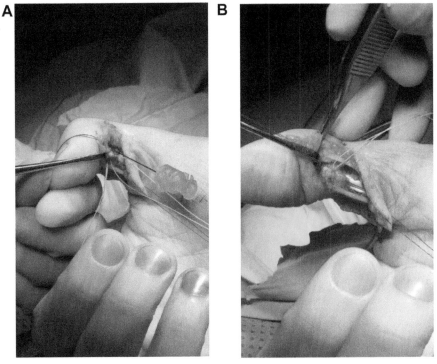

Fig. 8. Intraoperative photograph of zone 1 flexor tendon repair: (*A*) 4-0 cruciate repair of distal end and (*B*) completion of the primary repair.

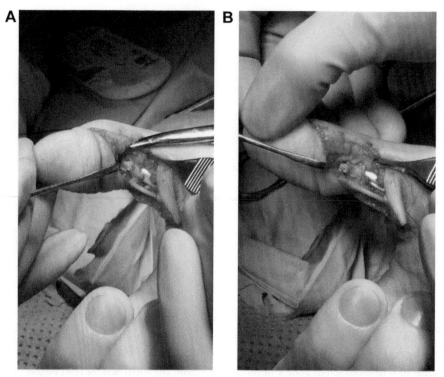

Fig. 9. Intraoperative photograph of zone 1 flexor tendon repair: (*A*) epitendinous repair using 5-0 prolene in mattress fashion in flexion and (*B*) extension.

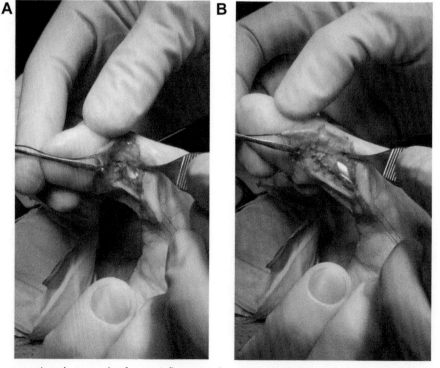

Fig. 10. Intraoperative photograph of zone 1 flexor tendon repair: evaluation of repair site with passive IPJ (*A*) flexion and (*B*) extension.

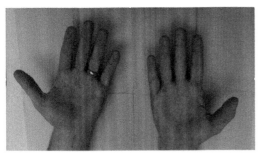

Fig. 11. Postoperative clinical photograph of zone 1 flexor tendon repair: resting position.

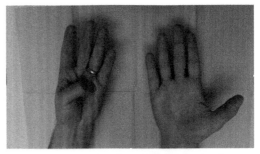

Fig. 13. Postoperative clinical photograph of zone 1 flexor tendon repair: active left thumb flexion.

- If the pullout technique is performed with a button or K-wire fixation, the suture or wires are removed at 8 weeks postsurgery.
- Strengthening exercises are initiated between 2 and 3 months postoperatively.

Case example 1: zone 1 flexor tendon laceration

A 33-year-old left-hand dominant gentleman presented with pain and stiffness of his right thumb. Two days before presentation, the patient was cutting a bagel when the knife slipped and punctured his right thumb. He noticed bleeding and pain. He presented to an Urgent Care facility the next day where the wound was irrigated and primarily closed. Ever since the injury, the patient has had inability to flex the right thumb at the IP joint.

Clinical examination was significant for a transverse laceration at the volar thumb just proximal to the IP joint with loss of IPJ flexion (**Fig. 3**) at rest and while active. There was strong suspicion for complete FPL laceration. Risks, benefits, alternatives, and complications of the procedure were discussed and the patient consented to surgery.

A midlateral incision was made at the volar aspect of the right thumb. On examination of the

FPL, it had been completely transected distal to the oblique pulley, and the proximal end was visualized in the wound with vinculae remaining (**Fig. 4**). The proximal end was stabilized using a 25-gauge hypodermic needle (**Fig. 5**), whereas the distal end was localized after confirming integrity of the oblique pulley (**Fig. 6**).

After tendon localization and stabilization, repair was begun using 3-0 ethibond suture in a 4-strand cruciate technique with the proximal (**Fig. 7**) than distal ends (**Fig. 8**). Epitendinous repair was performed using 5-0 Prolene in mattress fashion (**Fig. 9**) and the pulley preserved (see **Fig. 9**). Tracking of the repair was evaluated in flexion and extension at the IPJ (**Fig. 10**).

The patient was placed in a dorsal blocking splint, and therapy consisting of early active range of motion was begun 3 days postoperatively.

Patient range of motion at time of final evaluation 3 months postoperatively demonstrated slight flexion contracture (15 degrees) and flexion similar to the contralateral side (**Figs. 11–14**, Video 1).

Case example 2: zone 1 flexor tendon avulsion, Leddy type II with distal phalanx fracture

A 50-year-old right-hand dominant woman presented with left small finger pain and stiffness after

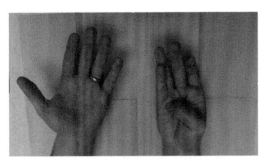

Fig. 12. Postoperative clinical photograph of zone 1 flexor tendon repair: active right thumb flexion.

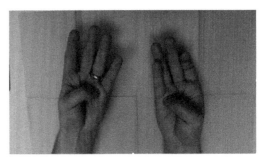

Fig. 14. Postoperative clinical photograph of zone 1 flexor tendon repair: comparison view of bilateral active thumb flexion.

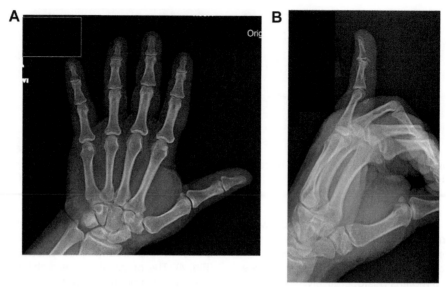

Fig. 15. Preoperative clinical (*A*) PA and (*B*) lateral radiographs of zone 1 flexor tendon avulsion injury.

her dog's leash twisted it 3 days before presentation. Clinical examination was significant for swelling and impaired flexion at the right small finger at the DIP joint. Radiographic evaluation was significant for right small finger flexor avulsion with avulsion fragment as well as distal phalanx fracture, Leddy type II (**Fig. 15**). Risks, benefits, alternatives, and complications of the procedure were discussed and the patient consented to surgery.

A Bruner-style incision was made at the volar aspect of the right small finger (**Fig. 16**). On

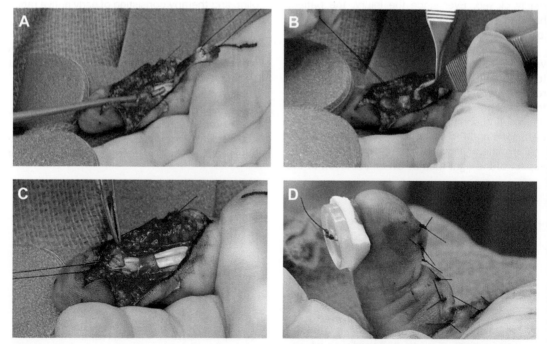

Fig. 16. Intraoperative photographs of zone 1 flexor tendon avulsion repair: (*A*) A4 pulley dilation. (*B*) Atraumatic passage of FDP through A4 pulley using tagging sutures. (*C*) Completed passage of FDP tendon. (*D*) Final repair using 2-0 PDS and suture button.

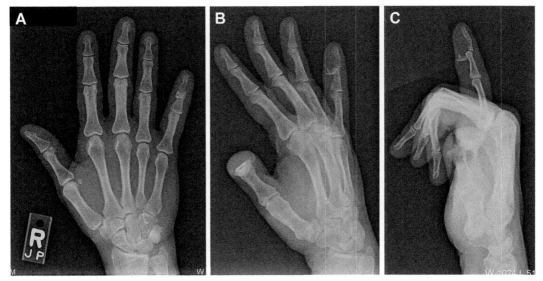

Fig. 17. Preoperative (*A*) PA and (*B*) oblique and (*C*) lateral radiographs of zone 1 flexor tendon avulsion injury.

examination of the FDP, it was attached to the volar distal phalanx fracture whereas the A4 pulley was intact. The A4 pulley was gently dilated using a rubber catheter.

3-0 ethibond sutures were placed in the proximal tendon end, and the tendon was rerouted underneath the A4 pulley in an atraumatic fashion using smooth forceps. A Keith needle was used to drill 2 holes through the remainder of the distal phalanx. 2-0 PDS was used to perform tendon-

bone repair, with the remaining suture passed through the holes to the dorsal nail. Repair was completed by tying the 2-0 PDS over a button to protect the nail. Additional 3-0 ethibond was used to augment the tendon-repair bone site.

The patient was placed in a dorsal blocking splint, and therapy consisting of early active range of motion was initiated. Sutures and the button were removed at 8 weeks postoperatively.

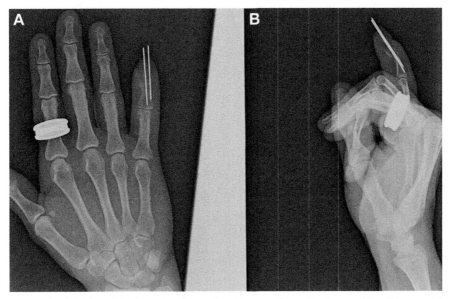

Fig. 18. Postoperative (*A*) PA and (*B*) lateral radiographs of zone 1 flexor tendon avulsion injury repaired using a combination of K-wires and suture fixation, week 6.

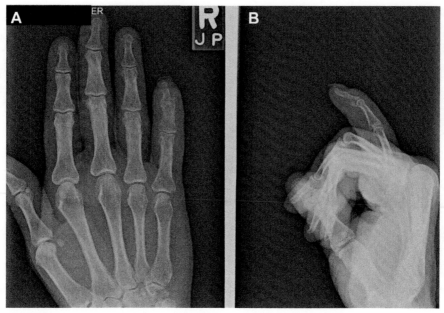

Fig. 19. Postoperative (*A*) PA and (*B*) lateral radiographs of zone 1 flexor tendon avulsion injury repaired using a combination of K-wires and suture fixation, week 8.

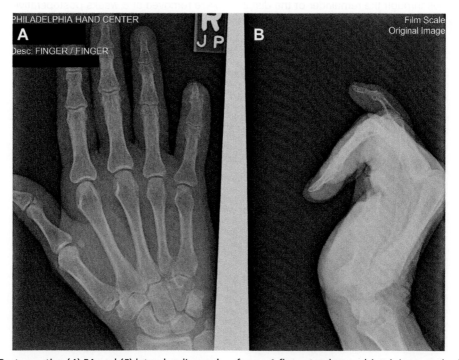

Fig. 20. Postoperative (*A*) PA and (*B*) lateral radiographs of zone 1 flexor tendon avulsion injury repaired using a combination of K-wires and suture fixation, week 12.

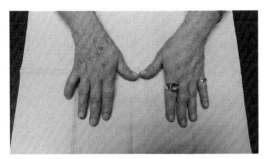

Fig. 21. Postoperative clinical photographs of zone 1 flexor tendon avulsion injury repair. Resting position.

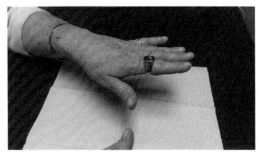

Fig. 23. Postoperative clinical photographs of zone 1 flexor tendon avulsion injury repair. Left-hand extension.

Case example 3: zone 1 flexor tendon avulsion, Leddy type V

A 51-year-old right-hand dominant woman presented with right small finger pain and stiffness after someone twisted it significantly. Clinical examination was significant for tenting of the skin and impaired flexion at the right small finger DIP joint. Radiographic evaluation was significant for right small finger flexor avulsion with avulsion fragment as well as distal phalanx fracture, Leddy type V (see **Fig. 16**). Risks, benefits, alternatives, and complications of the procedure were discussed and the patient consented to surgery.

A Bruner-style incision was made at the volar aspect of the right small finger. On examination of the FDP, it was partially attached to the volar distal phalanx fracture and was completely displaced and rotated. The dorsal remaining distal phalanx was fractured and unstable.

Using two 0.035 K-wires, the distal phalanx fracture was reduced and fixed in a retrograde fashion across the IP joint.

The FDP tendon was repaired using 3-0 Ethibond fashion with 4 locking sutures.

The patient was placed in a dorsal blocking splint, and therapy consisting of active proximal interphalangeal joint and metacarpophalangeal joint range of motion was begun. The patient was minimally compliant with therapy.

Healing was evaluated 6 weeks after fixation (**Fig. 17**), and the pins were pulled.

Radiographic evaluation 8 weeks after surgery revealed increased bone healing (**Fig. 18**) and bone remodeling at time of final evaluation (**Figs. 19** and **20**).

Patient range of motion at time of final evaluation demonstrated slight flexion contracture (15 degrees) and flexion similar to the contralateral side (**Figs. 21–25**, Video 2).

OUTCOMES

Historically, laceration and avulsion injuries to zone 1 resulted in fair to poor results.[16,17] In the largest study of zone 1 primary flexor tendon repairs to date, Moiemen and Elliott examined outcomes in 102 patients undergoing surgery for zone 1 laceration (1a, 1b, and 1c) as well as avulsion (p).[9] In their assessment of the effects of these injuries on DIP joint motion alone, good-to-excellent results were obtained in only 50%, 46%, 50%, and 22%, respectively. More recently, other studies reviewed have

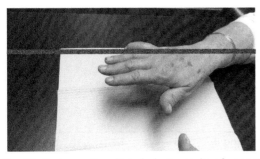

Fig. 22. Postoperative clinical photographs of zone 1 flexor tendon avulsion injury repair. Right-hand extension.

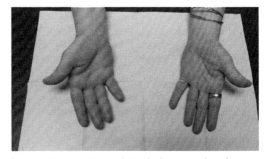

Fig. 24. Postoperative clinical photographs of zone 1 flexor tendon avulsion injury repair. Bilateral finger extension.

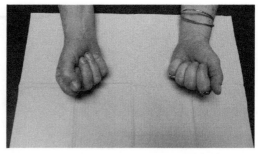

Fig. 25. Postoperative clinical photographs of zone 1 flexor tendon avulsion injury repair. Bilateral finger flexion.

documented approximately 80% excellent-to-good results, however with varied reports of DIP joint motion. A summary of the studies is outlined in **Table 2**.

The postoperative DASH score and DIP joint range of motion were reported inconsistently among various articles. Postoperatively, 71% of patients returned to work within 18 weeks.[22]

In the authors' experience, zone1 flexor tendon repairs pose unique challenges in that the (1) area of repair is small; (2) avulsion injuries require bone-to-bone healing, often of small fragments; (3) suture and wire/anchor techniques pose risk to the nail and development of nail injury; and (4) the likelihood for persistent postoperative flexion contracture at the DIP joint is high. Given these challenges, however, the possibility exists to obtain adequate postoperative DIP joint flexion and finger function with assiduous repair and therapy techniques.

Table 2
Summary of zone 1 primary flexor tendon repair studies to date

Author	Mechanism of Injury	Details	No. of Patients	%Good/ Excellent Results	DIP Joint ROM
Schaller & Baer,[18] 2010	Laceration	3-0 prolene suture and Kirchmayr technique with suture passing through distal tendon stump and exiting fingertip	65	95	NR
Zhang et al,[19] 2014	Avulsion	2 X 3-0 Ethibond sutures in a Becker configuration hold a 28-gauge steel wire that is passed dorsally through the distal phalanx and then secured to an externalized K-wire construct	16	81	8/32
Teo et al,[20] 2009	Laceration and avulsion	3-0 Ethibond passed through tendon using modified Kessler technique and then through drill holes at the sides of the distal phalanx with knot tied on volar surface of tendon	10	78	2.2/55.5
McCallister et al,[21] 2006	Laceration and avulsion	2 microbone anchors using 3-0 Ethibond and hemi-modified Kessler pattern	13	NR	8/56

Abbreviation: ROM, range of motion.

SUMMARY

A multitude of repair options are available to repair distal FDP tendon injuries depending on injury mechanism, chronicity, and patient-specific factors. Suture, wire, and anchor modes of fixation are used commonly to perform bone-to-tendon repairs. However, no technique is proved superior to others due to lack randomized trials and discrepancies in the outcome parameters studied by different investigators.

CLINICS CARE POINTS

- Patients with acute flexor tendon injuries should be treated within 1 week of injury if possible. Delay can result in adhesion formation and may reduce tendon excursion.
- Trimming the end of the tendon, if frayed or bulbous, may allow for easier passage through the sheath or pulley.
- Accurate tendon orientation is crucial.
- If the level of repair is close to the A4 pulley, the tendon must not be too bulky in order to glide through A4 easily. If there is difficulty, the distal aspect of A4 can be vented with a longitudinal incision without significant functional consequences.
- Care should be taken to avoid drilling into the nail base to prevent injury to the germinal matrix and possible nail deformity.
- For early motion therapy, use at least a 4-strand core suture technique with a running epitendinous suture.
- The tendon-bone junction site should be observed directly before final tying of the suture to ensure the tendon is making contact with cancellous bone at the repair site.
- Tendon advancement of more than 1 cm carries the risk of quadriga.[23]

DISCLOSURE

National Institutes of Health (RM).

SUPPLEMENTARY DATA

Supplementary data related to this article can be found online at https://doi.org/10.1016/j.hcl.2023.01.001.

REFERENCES

1. de Jong JP, Nguyen JT, Sonnema AJM, et al. The incidence of acute traumatic tendon injuries in the hand and wrist: a 10-year population-based study. Clin Orthop Surg 2014;6(2):196–202.
2. Leddy JP, Packer JW. Avulsion of the profundus tendon insertion in athletes. J Hand Surg 1977;2(1):66–9.
3. Manske PR, Lesker PA. Avulsion of the ring finger flexor digitorum profundus tendon: an experimental study. J Hand Surg Br Vol 1978;10(1):52–5.
4. Bynum DK, Gilbert JA. Avulsion of the flexor digitorum profundus: anatomic and biomechanical considerations. J Hand Surg 1988;13(2):222–7.
5. Kleinert HE, Kutz JE, Ashbell TS, Martinez E. Primary Repair of Lacerated Flexor Tendons in "No Man's Land." In: ; 2014.
6. Verdan CE. Half a century of flexor-tendon surgery. Current status and changing philosophies. J Bone Joint Surg Am 1972;54(3):472–91.
7. Ochiai N, Matsui T, Miyaji M, et al. Vascular anatomy of flexor tendons. I. Vincular system and blood supply of the profundus tendon in the digital sheath. J Hand Surg 1979;4(4):321–30.
8. Azar CA, Culver JE, Fleegler EJ. Blood supply of the flexor pollicis longus tendon. J Hand Surg Am 1983;8(4):471–5.
9. Moiemen NS, Elliot D. Primary flexor tendon repair in zone 1. J Hand Surg 2000;25B(1):78–84.
10. Fujihara Y, Ota H, Watanabe K. Utility of early active motion for flexor tendon repair with concomitant injuries: a multivariate analysis. Injury 2018;49(12):2248–51.
11. Higgins A, Lalonde DH, Bell M, et al. Avoiding flexor tendon repair rupture with intraoperative total active movement examination. Plast Reconstr Surg 2010;126(3):941–5.
12. Wade PJ, Wetherell RG, Amis AA. Flexor tendon repair: significant gain in strength from the Halsted peripheral suture technique. J Hand Surg Edinb Scotl 1989;14(2):232–5.
13. Huq S, George S, De B. Zone 1 flexor tendon injuries: a review of the current treatment options for acute injuries. J Plast Reconstr Aesthetic Surg 2013;66(8). https://doi.org/10.1016/j.bjps.2013.04.026.
14. Schreuder FB, Scougall PJ, Puchert E, et al. The effect of mitek anchor insertion angle to attachment of FDP avulsion injuries. J Hand Surg 2006;31(3):292–5.
15. Lee SK, Fajardo M, Kardashian G, et al. Repair of flexor digitorum profundus to distal phalanx: a biomechanical evaluation of four techniques. J Hand Surg 2011;36(10):1604–9.
16. Evans RB. A study of the zone 1 flexor tendon injury and implications for treatment. J Hand Ther 1990;133–48.
17. Gerbino PG, Saldana MJ, Westerbeck P, et al. Complications experienced in the rehabilitation of zone 1 flexor tendon injuries with dynamic splinting. J Hand Surg 1991;16A:680–6.

18. Schaller P, Baer W. Motion-stable flexor tendon repair with the Mantero technique in the distal part of the fingers. J Hand Surg Eur 2010;35(1):51–5.

19. Zhang X, Shao X, Zhang K. Pull-out wire traction for the treatment of avulsion of the flexor digitorum profundus from its insertion. J Hand Surg Eur 2014; 39(6):667–9.

20. Teo TC, Dionyssiou D, Armenio A, et al. Anatomical repair of zone 1 flexor tendon injuries. Plast Reconstr Surg 2009;123(2):617–22.

21. McCallister WV, Ambrose HC, Katolik LI, et al. Comparison of pullout button versus suture anchor for zone I flexor tendon repair. J Hand Surg 2006; 31(2):246–51.

22. Brady C, Lee A, Gardiner M, et al. The outcomes of zone 1 flexor digitorum profundus tendon injury: a systematic review and meta-analysis. J Plast Reconstr Aesthetic Surg 2022;75(2):893–939.

23. Gillig JD, Smith MD, Hutton WC, et al. The effect of flexor digitorum profundus tendon shortening on jersey finger surgical repair: a cadaveric biomechanical study. J Hand Surg Eur 2015;40(7): 729–34.

Printed and bound by CPI Group (UK) Ltd, Croydon, CR0 4YY

08/05/2025

01864717-0007